GOOD HEALTH GOD'S WAY

Living Healthy in an Unhealthy World

BY DALE BOYLL

Publisher's note:
Although the advice in this book is based on the author's extensive research, experience and counseling in nutrition, it is not intended to diagnose, prescribe, imply treatment or be a substitute for the advice of your personal physician.

Published by Scriptural Nutrition Press
P.O. Box 3085, Spring Hill, Florida 34611

2 4 6 8 10 9 7 5 3 1

ISBN: 0-9669720-0-7

Library of Congress
Catalog Card Number: 99-93599

Good Health God's Way: living healthy in an unhealthy world,
Dale Boyll author

Copy editor: Robert Hicks
Book design and production: Rudolph King Studios
Digital photo-illustration for cover: Craig Rudolph King

Healthy Cells

Of course, there are many things that contribute to healthy cells, and it is far beyond our scope here to even name them all, let alone explain them all. So, just one important factor will be discussed—the sodium-potassium pump.

Body cells are always struggling to obtain the right minerals and expel the wrong ones.

Body cells are always struggling to obtain the right minerals and expel the wrong ones. The "good" minerals for inside the cells are potassium and magnesium, while the "bad" minerals are sodium and calcium. High levels of potassium and magnesium in our cells are needed for the normal cell functions of energy production, protein manufacture, growth, repair, etc. But high levels of sodium and calcium depress these activities. When the imbalance gets bad enough the cell dies.

In normal healthy circumstances our cells easily maintain the proper ratio of minerals by pumping the good ones in and pumping the bad ones out. This pumping activity is necessary because without it, all of the minerals have a tendency to diffuse equally both inside and outside of the cells. Body cells spend a considerable amount of energy on this pumping activity.

Most free radicals have an affinity for the fatty acid membrane of our cell walls.

What typically happens in our modern western society is that free radical damage occurs in the cell wall. Most free radicals have an affinity for the fatty acid membrane of our cell walls. So, as free radicals overcome our antioxidant defenses the cells are weakened and begin to "leak". That is, potassium and magnesium leak out faster than they can be pumped back in, while sodium and calcium leak in faster than they can be pumped out. This is really bad news for the cell! One major reason why it is so bad is because the mitochondria (the little organelles that produce energy in the cell) require high levels of potassium and magnesium and cannot tolerate much sodium or calcium. So, just at the time that more energy is needed for more pumping, less energy is available. This is a vicious cycle that leads to cell malfunction and death. When the affected cells are in our joints we might get arthritis.

When they are in our kidneys we might get high blood pressure. When they are in our arteries we might have a stroke or heart attack. When they are—oh, you get the idea.

Free Radicals and Cardio-Vascular Disease.

Because more people die from arterial related disorders, let's use it as an example of how free radical damage could be the underlying cause of these diseases.

When a blood clot forms in an artery full of atherosclerotic plaque it is likely to get stuck in the artery

The cells, making up the lining on the inside of our blood vessels are sensitive to free-radical damage. Since our circulatory system is the major transportation system in our bodies, it is easy to see why free radicals would be there in large numbers. As the cells making up the lining of our arteries are damaged by free radicals the body naturally tries to protect them by covering them. This covering is similar to a scab that forms on a wound on our skin. This covering is composed of tough, fatty plaque containing a high percentage of cholesterol that we have been taught is the cause of atherosclerosis. However, rather than being the cause of atherosclerosis, this "gunk" seems to be the result of it. As these free radical-induced injuries are repeated, millions of times over many years, the rate of plaque buildup is faster than the rate of healing, and advanced atherosclerosis is the result.

Free Radicals Affect the Blood.

There are three main types of cells that make up our blood: 1) the red blood cells which carry oxygen to all cells in our body and carry carbon dioxide, a major waste product of metabolism, to our lungs for elimination, 2) White blood cells or lymphocytes which are a part of our immune system, and 3) Platelets which are used to repair a hole or cut, or a severed blood vessel.

One of the effects of free radical damage to red blood cells is that they become inflexible, unable to bend and fold. This is really bad because our smallest blood vessels, called capillaries, are only 4 microns in diameter while a red blood cell is about 7 microns wide. In normal circulation the red blood cells must fold in order to fit into the tiny capillaries. It makes for a tight squeeze that allows for excellent transference of oxygen and carbon dioxide. As more and more red blood cells become inflexible they are not able to fit into the capillaries thus depriving our cells of oxygen and the removal of waste products. Of course, oxygen is necessary for cell energy production and normal cell activity. Under-oxygenated cells quickly become weak and malfunction, leading to degenerative disease.

Severe free radical damage can cause red blood cells to rupture and release free iron and copper which can cause still more free radical activity and chain reactions. (We will discuss iron overload a little later in this chapter).

Circulating in the blood are a type of cell called platelets. Platelets help stop bleeding when vessels are broken or damaged. Large numbers of platelets stick together to plug-up a hole in the vessel. In a normal, healthy body these platelets don't stick together unless there is a "leak". When a leak occurs, certain hormones called prostaglandins increase the stickiness of the platelets so they will stick together and plug the leak.

Under free radical attack platelets can stick together when there is no hole to be plugged. This process is called thrombosis and the mass of sticky platelets is called a thrombus or blood clot. When a blood clot forms in an artery full of atherosclerotic plaque (or if a piece of the plaque breaks away and becomes a thrombus), it is likely to get stuck in the artery, blocking or reducing the flow of blood. When this happens in a coronary artery it causes a heart attack. When it happens in the brain it causes a stroke.

You might have heard that an aspirin or two a day improves circulation and may help prevent thrombosis and therefore heart attacks and strokes. Aspirin does this by inhibiting the formation and effectiveness of prostaglandins. Aspirin thereby inhibits platelet stickiness and thins the blood for better circulation. The trouble is prostaglandins are important for other functions of our body. For example, prostaglandins play a role in certain immune system functions. The kidneys need prostoglandins to perform their filtering and cleansing work. When prostaglandins are inhibited, kidneys have a hard time doing their work. In fact, there is strong scientific evidence that aspirin and similar drugs can cause kidney damage. Also, everyone agrees that aspirin can cause digestive system problems including stomach and duodenal ulcers.

Where We Get Free Radicals

Incomplete Digestion. There are many contributing factors to digestive system disorders which lead to incomplete digestion of food and free radical formation. However, we almost always bring these things upon ourselves by the choices we make. One problem is eating a disproportionally high ratio of certain foods like fats.

Polyunsaturated fats are tremendously effective promoters of free radical damage. So much, in fact, that scientific researchers have found it easier and more reliable to simply add polyunsaturates to the diet than to ensure that the animals are deficient in antioxidants.

Saturated fats are somewhat more stable than polyunsaturates, but are still very susceptible to oxidation. This is a big problem, especially with fatty meats that are ground or processed and heated. In other words, by the time that hamburger or other ground meat is cooked, it'll be dripping with free radical producing oxidized fats and cholesterol. Processed meats like hot dogs and bologna are laced with chemical preservatives like nitrites that add fuel to the free radical fire. In addition, when nitrites are eaten they combine with humic acid (a naturally occurring substance in our body) to form nitrosamine. Nitrosamine is the very chemical that many research scientists use to cause cancer in laboratory animals.

One of the worst problems in our dietary choices is the lack of sufficient dietary fiber. The average American eats less than one third of the fiber they need to maintain good digestion and promote health. Still another big contributor to incomplete digestion is the overuse of antibiotics, both in human consumption and feeding it to our meat animals; beef, poultry, etc. Antibiotics disrupt the flora in our digestive tract allowing toxins and poisons to form and be taken up by our portal vein system and deposited directly into our liver. For a better understanding of digestion read Chapter 7.

The average American eats less than one third of the fiber they need to maintain good digestion and promote health

Chemical pollutants in our air, water and food as well as pharmaceuticals contribute to free radicals and are discussed later in some detail.

Synthetic nutrients and inappropriate ratios of vitamins and minerals.

This area of discussion is going to be a real eye opener. For many, it is an area that they have never really considered before. Many elements which are generally desirable (nutrients) can accumulate in excess and cause free radical pathology. Also, certain combinations of nutrients when in excess or the wrong ratios will turn destructive. We will discuss just two examples that fit in readily with our discussions, but please remember, there are hundreds of nutrients and nearly an infinite number of nutrient combinations.

Vitamin D - The Sunshine Vitamin.

As most of you know, vitamin D is called the Sunshine vitamin because it is made in our bodies when sunshine striking our skin helps change cholesterol into vitamin D. Perhaps you didn't know that it is much more like a hormone than a vitamin and as such has many detrimental effects when taken as a dietary supplement rather than using the natural pathway of production—sunshine.

It has been known for many years that supplementation of Vitamin D causes heart attacks in experimental animals. Recent studies have confirmed this and offered as a reason the fact that excess Vitamin D causes a magnesium deficiency in cells, particularly heart cells. Do you remember that magnesium is one of the "good" minerals for the inside of cells? Vitamin D has been identified long ago as an angiotoxic substance, that is, a substance that irritates the lining of blood vessels. We now know that the source of that irritation is free radical damage.

Over the years, many individuals and organizations have recommended that vitamin D, NOT be supplementally added to our foods. Yet today an increasing array of foods are fortified with Vitamin D. Foods like milk, dairy products, baby foods, some beverages, sauces, breakfast cereals, margarine, macaroni, noodles, flour and many others. It is estimated that the average American gets 5 to 8 times more Vitamin D than they need.

Just two more points about Vitamin D. Remember, Vitamin D is more like a hormone and we shouldn't consistently eat hormones. Many studies have been done to show that naturally produced Vitamin D through exposure to sunlight is always healthful and never toxic.

Iron

Iron and other nutritionally essential metals can cause oxidant stress when present in excess. Iron is the most important since it has much more potential for causing free radical pathology and it is much easier to obtain and retain an excess of it. The amount of iron is not the only consideration. The type of iron is important, whether it is organic or inorganic, if it is chelated or not, and whether it is decompartmentalized all play a part in whether iron in our bodies is good for us or not. Another factor is the relative ratios of other nutrients present.

For example, the combination of ascorbic acid (Vitamin C) with free iron is a very powerful cause of free radical pathology. Scientists often use ascorbic acid with iron to induce free radical pathology, and to study the protective effects of antioxidants against that pathology. That doesn't mean that the proper amount of iron and vitamin C is bad. It's not! It's only when we get out of balance that there is a problem.

Iron Overload

Regular indulgence in deep fat, fried foods is a sure recipe for free radical damage, accelerated aging and disease.

Accumulation of excess iron in the body is very possible. Your body is extremely iron efficient, retaining and recycling it over and over again. In fact, there is no normal mechanism for removing iron from the system. The body's iron level is controlled by absorption and can build up with dietary increases. This is especially true of men.

For many years it was thought that premenopausal women were protected from heart disease by their female hormones. These hormones were used in an attempt to prevent and treat heart disease but the results were poor and the side effects very great. Then researchers found that people with heart disease have high iron levels and younger women don't. The obvious correlation is that women release a lot of iron in their monthly menstrual flow. And here we thought that the centuries old practice of blood letting was antiquated, barbaric and unscientific!

One combination which causes a lot of damage is iron and fat. All foods contain iron chelating proteins which prevent the iron from coming in contact with the fats in that food. These proteins actually protect the fat from the potentially harmful iron. Many of these proteins are destroyed during food processing, especially in meats. Of course they are completely absent from iron supplements.

Iron in contact with fats greatly speed up free radical reactions. Unbound iron is a potent catalyst of free radical chain reactions especially in injured cells and tissues. Oxidation of food fats proceed much too rapidly when free iron is available. Deep fat fried foods are the worst. Regular indulgence in deep fat fried foods is a sure recipe for free radical damage, accelerated aging and disease.

The absorption of iron from plant foods is regulated by phytates. Phytates are part of those phytonutrients found in abundance in all vegetable foods that scientists are just beginning to understand. Certain phytates allow iron and other metals to be absorbed, but only if the body needs them. If the body already has plenty of iron, then the phytates tend to depress further absorption.

One pitfall is that many antioxidants are capable, under certain conditions, of acting as pro-oxidants.

If our major source of iron was plants, there would be almost no chance of iron overload. However, Americans eat a lot of iron rich red meats (meats with the blood still in it), we fortify many foods with extra iron and we use a lot of supplementary iron and Vitamin C which greatly enhances iron absorption.

Meat contains iron in the form of heme, (as in hemoglobin) which is much easier to absorb than iron from vegetables. Heme iron is absorbed regardless of need because phytates do not depress the absorption of heme iron. In fact, heme iron enhances the absorption of non-heme iron.

We add iron to most of the processed grain foods like flour and cereals, while removing the phytates. The result is four times more iron absorption of inorganic iron with high doses of Vitamin C which can lead to iron overload and free radical damage. Add to all of this a lot of free iron in our drinking water, and it is not hard to see why iron overload can be a major contributing factor in free radical pathology, especially for men.

Antioxidants to the Rescue?

With all the problems with free radical production and damage we have naturally turned to antioxidants as the solution. This seems logical and desirable, but is it?

Unfortunately, antioxidants may have very dangerous, unwanted side effects. Antioxidants may not be selective and may blunt a number of normally occurring, life supporting free radical reactions such as are found in mitochondrial electron transport (energy production), in prostaglandin synthesis, in phagocytic leucocytes (immune function) and other processes. Many antioxidants are also metal chelators and may adversely affect the synthesis and activity of several metal-dependent enzymes, including the superoxide dismutasis which are key free radical controlling enzymes.

Unfortunately, the use of immoderate quantities of nutrients is now a common practice!

One pitfall is that many antioxidants are capable under certain conditions of acting as pro-oxidants. For example, ascorbic acid has been glibly dubbed an antioxidant, but this property is concentration-dependent and is exerted only if some metals such as iron are absent. Another problem with many antioxidants is their metal chelating properties. If we are loaded with antioxidants that have chelating abilities, it is possible to disarray the entire copper/zinc/manganese ratios and decrease SOD activities.

Wow! That makes antioxidants sound awfully dangerous. Of course, natural antioxidants under normal conditions are not dangerous, they are extremely healthful. Only the uninformed and foolish use of immoderate quantities of nutritional antioxidants or the misguided use of synthetic antioxidants are dangerous.

Unfortunately, the use of immoderate quantities of nutrients is now a common practice! There is a relatively new field in nutrition science called nutritional pharmacology (also known as "mega-vitamin therapy"). Nutritional pharmacology is the study of drug-like effects of nutrients when used in much larger amounts than usual, or simply the use of nutrients as drugs. Just because a substance happens to be a nutrient does not mean that it is free from potential hazards. The field of nutritional pharmacology has much more to do with pharmacology than to nutrition. The "*if a little is good, more must be better*" approach may be harmless with whole foods, but not with the drug/supplements that are available today.

It is quite common for a person to go into a health food store, read a one page write-up about a vitamin, hormone, mineral, amino acid, or other "nutrient" and then overdose on it. After all it's "natural" and needed and the write-up made it sound like just the thing to overcome a problem.

As an example, read the following paragraph:

"Niacin is required for the formation of a coenzyme called NADPH that is depleted by oxidant stress. NADPH is involved in maintaining the activity of the antioxidant enzyme glutathione peroxidase. Riboflavin is needed by another enzyme, glutathione reductase, that is responsible for recycling glutathione after it has been oxidized by glutathione peroxidase, thus, both niacin and riboflavin are essential for this antioxidant activity."

Why don't we just do it God's way?

Sounds like we need lots of those two B vitamins, doesn't it?

But, now read the next paragraph:

"Niacin and riboflavin activate oxidizing enzymes which produce free radicals. Xanthine oxidase, for example, is activated by riboflavin and iron. NADPH stimulates iron catalyzed free radical generation. Niacin has produced elevations of blood enzyme levels suggesting liver damage caused by free radical pathology."

Both paragraphs are true so what do we do? *Everyone agrees* that we need just the right amount of just the proper kinds of all our nutrients and then we will be healthy. That's where agreement ends and controversy begins. NO two "authorities" seem to agree on the "right" amount or the "proper" kinds, not to mention their relative ratios. And we have considered just a few vitamins, minerals, enzymes and hormones. Can you imagine the confusion if we would try to take into consideration all the vitamins, all the minerals, all the enzymes, all the hormones, all the neurotransmitters, all of the waste products, all the viruses, all kinds of bacteria, all environmental toxins, all genetic factors, all emotional stress and everything else that effects our health? Do you really think human kind is ever going to figure it all out? Why don't we just do it God's way?

Simply put, God's way requires obedience to God's laws (suggestions for our healthy living) and mankind has never been very obedient to God. All the confusion and controversy about nutrition and health shouldn't really be too surprising. In 2 Timothy 4:3-4, Paul tells us, "For the time will come when men will not put up with sound doctrine. Instead, to suit their own desires, they will gather around them a great number of teachers to say what their itching ears want to hear. They will turn their ears away from the truth and turn aside to myths."

Don't you believe that it is man's desire to eat whatever tastes good, to drink whatever makes them feel good, to take whatever they want? Why else do we eat so much sugar and fat? Why else do we drink so much alcohol? Why else do we smoke so many cigarettes, abuse so many drugs and indulge in every kind of gluttony? Why else?

God's way is so much simpler and so much better. We don't have to "figure it out", because God has already figured it out. God not only figured it all out but He wrote it down for us. He put everything we need to build and rebuild our bodies in our food. For about 1700 years or so our food was fruits, vegetables, seeds, grains and nuts. Then He added meats to our diet. But He also told us which meats were good for us and which meats were unhealthy for us. He gave us many other suggestions for our well being and good health. Things like...don't eat blood, don't eat fat, don't worry, don't let the sun go down on your anger, forgive everybody, etc. Think about this. We cannot break God's laws, we only break ourselves over them.

THE PROBLEM & THE SOLUTION

THE PROBLEM: The overall health in America is declining, not getting better. Some people might disagree. Take a look at the major killers in Chapter 6.

ANOTHER PROBLEM: Most disease is caused by malnutrition and/or poisoning. If the body had the building blocks it needed in sufficient quantity and at the right time and place, in the absence of too many toxins and poisons, it would overcome disease.

THREE POSSIBLE ANSWERS:

1. **Simply eat natural wholesome foods instead of processed, refined, artificial foods.** This is a step in the right direction, but won't overcome all the problems. Most foods Americans can buy don't have the nutrients they should because of depleted soils, chemicals used, picking unripened produce, shipping long distances, processing, refining, etc.
2. **Supplement with vitamins and minerals.** This might help a little, but nearly all vitamins sold in the U.S. are synthetic chemical isolates and have limited vitamin activity in the body, and as we have seen, can be very destructive. See chapter on Vitamins.
3. **Modern Medical Science will heal me.** Most people rely on their doctor but let's look at the facts. Since the 'War on Cancer' was declared in 1971, billions of dollars have been spent to cure that dreaded disease. During that time deaths from cancer have more than doubled, and are at an all time high. According to the Center for Disease Control, 700,000 people a year die from medical treatment.

THE REAL SOLUTION: Follow the rules for healthy living laid down in the Bible. The Bible tells us what is good to eat and what is not good to eat. It tells us how to farm, the importance of sanitation and how to avoid disease. In fact, the Bible addresses every aspect of living. **It's doing it God's way!**

There are very few companies that make health products in line with these high principles.

WORDS TO KNOW

Free Radical

Antioxidant

Oxidation

Mitochondria

Atherosclerosis

Prostaglandins

Enzymes

SUMMARY

1. Free radicals are the underlying phsyical cause of most of our degenerative health problems today.
2. We get free radicals from incomplete digestion, polluted air, water and food, pharmaceuticals, fat and synthetic nutrients.
3. Our body's antioxidant defenses are our free radical fighters.
4. Our antioxidant defenses suffer because of bad farming methods, over-processed foods, wrong food choices, stressful lifestyles and inappropriate supplementation.
5. Free radicals affect every system of our bodies. For example, free radicals cause plaque to form on the inside of our arteries and cause blood clots.
6. Many times nutrients can be destructive. For example, too much iron and ascorbic acid cause free radicals.
7. The correct solution is balanced nutrition from "real" food—doing it God's way.

2

OUR DECLINING HEALTH PICTURE

PROVERBS 19:3

A man's own folly ruins his life, yet his heart rages against the Lord.

Many people today are afraid that the United States is losing her greatness. To those people I would like to point out that the U.S. leads the world in many important areas, like colon cancer, heart disease, diabetes, arthritis, and mental illness. We have more doctors, the finest hospitals, and spend more money for health care per capita than any other country; yet we are far from the healthiest nation on earth.

Around the turn of the century the United States was number one in world health. What has gone wrong? What is causing the plague of degenerative diseases that are killing our people both young and old? Several years ago Dr. Theodore Cooper — Assistant Secretary for Health for the Department of H.E.W. said, "There appears to be general agreement that the kinds and amount of food and beverages we consume and the style of living common in our generally affluent, sedentary society may be the major factors associated with the cause of cardiovascular disease, cancer and other chronic illnesses." In other words, what we eat and the way we live make us sick!

Let's take a look at some of the differences between life style and eating habits of the 1990's as compared to, let's say, 1900. Many of our great grandparents lived and worked on a farm with plenty of exercise, sunshine and fresh air. Grandma reared the kids, grew a garden, baked the bread and cooked the meals. By-in-large, our great grandparents ate fresh agricultural products. Today only 5% live on a farm, the wife must work in an office or factory to make ends meet, kids are raised in day care centers and we eat in fast food restaurants.

In 1900 we ate fresh, nutritious home-cooked meals. What do we put in our bodies today? Herbicides, fungicides, insecticides, pesticides, preservatives, artificial colors, artificial flavors, chemical additives, fluoride, chlorine, mercury, MSG, caffeine, nicotine, alcohol, medicines, drugs, carbon monoxide, X-rays and radiation. In general, processed, refined, chemicalized, dead foods. Then we chase them down with synthetic vitamins and expect to be healthy. God's laws don't work that way. Read the 28th Chapter of Deuteronomy and see if it doesn't sound like what has happened to us today.

Vibrant health should be more than the ability to walk down hill with the wind at your back!

Are you healthy? The answer might be found in your medicine cabinet; pain killers, antacids, tranquilizers, decongestants, anti-cough medicines, inhalers, nasal sprays, laxatives, sedatives, diet pills, etc., etc. Vibrant health should be more than the ability to walk down hill with the wind at your back.

Cancer, heart disease, allergies, ulcers, arthritis and diabetes have all increased greatly in this century. There are many problem areas — i.e.: sugar. Yet the consumption of sugar continues to increase. The average American now eats one hundred and sixty-seven pounds of sugar every year. Sugar gives you nothing except a sweet taste and empty calories! A bowl of oatmeal has 87 calories and is packed with vitamins, minerals, enzymes and fiber. A Danish pastry has 275 calories and is devoid of nutrients. Which would you rather have? What do you give your kids?

It is estimated that 56% of the American diet is artificial food. Let's take a look at breakfast for example: there is artificial juice, artificial eggs, artificial bacon (it is probably better to eat that than swine flesh), artificial bread (one can't call white flour food any more than they can call cocaine food), artificial butter, artificial jam, artificial coffee, artificial sugar, artificial cream, and of course, artificial vitamins. None of these so called foods have many nutrients and none of them have any "life force". What is meant by life force? If you take a grain of wheat and plant it in the ground it will grow and produce more wheat. The thing that caused the wheat to grow is life force. That's what we need to eat to maintain good health; live foods, not dead, processed foods.

Don't let anyone fool you. Our lifestyle and dietary habits DO determine our health — good or bad.

The Bible tells us very early what to eat. Take a look at the Original Bible Diet at the end of this chapter. If you ate that way you would be getting about 70% of your caloric intake as complex carbohydrates, 15% protein and 15% fat, plus a huge bonus of a great variety of dietary fiber. However, most of us get 3 to 5 times more protein and fat than is good for us, loads of **"empty calories"** in sugars, while we are only getting 25 to 30% of the needed complex carbohydrates and fiber.

THE PROPER PATH TO HEALTH

Narrow is the path that leads to health, broad is the road that leads to disease. Unfortunately, these statements are true, particularly in our Western society. Not because the principles of good health have changed. They have remained exactly the same for thousands of years. But our world has changed dramatically in recent decades and the rate of change continues to escalate. Changes in our thinking, our philosophy, our knowledge and our environment are happening so rapidly that we simply can't keep up!

Our bodies have been designed to work in certain ways and that IS the way it works. Nothing is going to change that, not our thinking, not our philosophy, not our knowledge, NOTHING! For example, our bodies have been designed to eat food, but modern scientific thinking says we can thrive on chemicals. We can't! So, this thinking is one lane in that broad highway that leads to disease.

The proper path to health and indeed, all aspects of life, should be based entirely on Godly principles. Your body knows how to build and rebuild itself given the proper building blocks and tools (nutrients) in a clean environment (not too many toxins and poisons).

The choice is crystal clear for those who are willing to seek and admit to truth. Follow the proven principles that will glorify God and lead to health and success.

Mad Cow Disease was caused by feeding cows to cows.

LEARNING FROM COWS

Have you ever heard the term bovine spongiform encephalopathy? It's also known as BSE or simply 'mad cow disease'. This disease is brand new. It first came on the scene in 1986. At first no one thought it was serious, but in the last few years, in Britain, over one million cows have been destroyed because of BSE. That's not the worst part; several dozen people have also died from the disease. Not to mention hundreds of domestic cats and other animals.

In 1996 the Center of Disease Control, the World Health Organization and the British government all concluded that 'mad cow disease' was caused by feeding cows to cows. This cannibalistic feeding practice first started in the 1950's and has been common practice for over 20 years in Europe and America. Oh, they make it sound innocent enough, calling this "feed" protein concentrates. It's made up of contaminated dairy products, internal organs from slaughterhouses, blood, and the carcases of diseased and dead cattle and other animals. All of these waste products are taken to rendering plants where they are cooked down into cattle feed. The end product resembles brown sugar. Incidentally ladies, a lot of the fat is skimmed off and made into cosmetics such as lipstick.

Everyone always thought that the rendering process destroyed all possible disease causing agents, like bacteria, viruses, parasites, etc. But everyone was wrong! The disease causing agent in this case is something called a 'prion'. The prion is apparently indestructible because it is not alive, like a bacteria or a virus or a parasite is alive. At least science has not been able to find any nucleic acid (RNA or DNA) associated with it. A prion is simply a misshapen brain protein. It has all the parts of a normal brain protein but is shaped differently. This prion is infectious because it somehow has the ability to change a normal brain protein into its own abnormal shape. Deformed brain proteins then clump together leaving holes in the brain. Since the prion is chemically identical to the normal brain protein, our immune system is apparently unable to recognize them as foreign invaders. So the prion continues to do its damage year after year.

The worst scenarios estimate that from 10 million up to 32 million Britains will die from Mad Cow Disease.

Scientists now agree that the BSE prion can infect most other species including man. The first human case was in Britain in 1994. How many people in Britain will die from 'mad cow disease'? As always, scientists vary widely in their estimates. The best scenarios project between 10,000 and 100,000 deaths. The worst scenarios estimate that from 10 million up to 32 million Britains will die from BSE. Even if the worst happens we probably won't see large numbers of deaths until 2005 or so.

Scientists believe that it will take about 20 years for the average infected person to die from BSE. Can you imagine the suffering of the victims and their families as the brain disintegrates affecting every part of the person's body and personality?

IS AMERICAN BEEF SAFE?

The FDA finally prohibited American cattlemen and meat packers from feeding cows to cows in June, 1997. However, this FDA ruling specifically exempts rendered poultry, horses and pigs as well as gelatin, blood and milk from the ban. So, even if this new ruling can be enforced, cows can still get their protein concentrates. Just as a further point of information, did you know that it is common practice to feed chicken manure to cows? The point of this discussion is really quite simple. What are cows designed to eat?—feed made from animals and manure or grains and grasses? That question leads us to our final point. What are people designed to eat ?...food or chemicals?

HEALTH PARADIGM

Americans eat 1/3 of their meals in fast food restaurants.

When we are first introduced to a holistic approach to health such as is promoted in this book, we do not fully appreciate it because we have been brought up all our lives looking at health from our modern, western scientific point of view, a worldly point of view. Our training and our culture has embedded in our mind the correct, proper and acceptable things to do as they apply to our health. Do you agree that the following are correct, proper and acceptable things to do?:

1. Giving candy (a nutrient-free "food" source) to our kids as a reward, thus linking a detrimental dietary habit with love and caring.
2. Promoting sodas and colas (nutrient-free beverages with many harmful effects) as the most popular drink in America, available everywhere, anytime.
3. Eating one third of our meals in fast food restaurants even after we know these meals are extremely low in nutrient value but very high in salt, fat and sugar.
4. Not being responsible for our own health but expecting the doctor to 'cure' us when we get sick.

These and many other social mores influence our thinking to the point that we can not see these obvious wicked destructive forces. The medical establishment, the fast food industry, the huge drug companies and many other forces are such an integral part of our lives, provide so much of our income and so many jobs, that we are all dependent on "the system". Anywhere money is involved, we quickly develop a bias against anything that would threaten our income.

So, because of the way we have been brought up, our scientific training and our bias toward the system, all heavily contribute to the prevailing paradigm. Therefore, when a Godly approach that looks at health from a Biblical point of view is advocated, most Americans don't want to see it. Even those that are open minded and try to understand where the different approach is coming from have a difficult time seeing the holistic picture. Let's use an understandable example. It would be hard for an avid football fan born and reared in Green Bay, Wisconsin to become a Chicago Bear's fan.

After we ourselves have decided to glorify God in all that we do, even including our dietary habits, it is very easy to become frustrated or even annoyed with people who don't. Never let that happen! But always be prepared to correct and encourage with great patience and careful instruction.

THE ORIGINAL BIBLE DIET

(Genesis 1:29)

"And God said. Behold, I have given you every herb bearing seed, which is upon the face of all the earth, and every tree, in which the fruit of a tree yielding seed: to you it shall be for meat."

Behold, I have given you every herb bearing seed... (a seed which does not develop wood-persistent tissue). Some examples are:

GRAINS: Wheat, corn, rye, barley, rice, millet, oats, and buckwheat.

SEEDS: Sunflower, sesame, flax, and pumpkinseeds etc.

LEGUMES: Soybeans, lentils, peas, peanuts, other beans.

SUCCULENT FOODS (containing seeds): Eggplant, okra, bell pepper, squash, green beans, pumpkins, cucumbers, tomatoes, and melons.

"*...and every tree, in which the fruit of a tree yielding seed...*" This category is the woody, perennial plants, shrubs, or bushes. Some examples are:

FRUIT TREES: Citrus fruits, sub-acid fruits, sweet fruits, neutral fruits.

NUTS: Almonds, pecans, cashews, brazil, walnuts, chestnuts, filberts, acorns, and pine nuts.

"*...TO YOU IT SHALL BE FOR MEAT.*"

Originally the green herbs were given by God as food for the animals. (Genesis 1:30).

"And to every BEAST of the earth, and to every Fowl of the air. and to everyTHING that creepeth upon the earth... I have given every GREEN HERB for MEAT: and it was so."

But. these vegetables (green herbs) were added to man's diet after he sinned (to help fight disease), and are a part of our diet today.

"And unto Adam He said. Because thou hast harkened unto the voice of thy wife... cursed is the ground for thy sake... and thou SHALT EAT the HERB of the Field." (Genesis 3:17, 18)

Some of these VEGETABLES include:

LEAFY HERBS: Celery, Cabbage, Kale, Chard, Lettuce, etc.

FLOWERS: Globe Artichoke, Broccoli, Cauliflower.

ROOTS: Carrots, Beets, Potatoes,Turnips, etc.

SUMMARY

1. America's level of health continues to decline.
2. The Bible tells us what to eat.
3. The holistic approach to good health follows scriptural principles.
4. The philosophy of regeneration is in line with these scriptural principles.
5. When we learn something from our youth, it is hard to see it any other way.

3

CHOICES AND HABITS

If a person suffering on his death bed was offered one month of illness-free, pain-free, vibrant life to be with his family, to make right some wrong he had done, to go some place he always wanted to go or do something that he always wanted to do, would he accept? Would you accept under those circumstances? What if you had to give up smoking, eat right for that month, forgive everyone and pay $250.00? Would you accept then? Most people would accept it in a heartbeat and consider it a very small price to pay!

PROVERBS 2:20:

In the house of the wise are stores of choice food and oil, but a foolish man devours all he has.

In real, everyday life we are all given exactly that choice every month! Unfortunately it is usually no longer available to a person on their death bed. Typically, most people mortgage their future. Some because of ignorance. Some in defiance. Some because of depression and apathy. All with the same joy-robbing and life-shortening effect.

We were created in God's image to be overcomers. Some say that we were born to suffer; that even as Christ suffered, so must we suffer. That's partially true, but there is a big difference between suffering abuse from the world because we will not deny our belief in God and His Son, our Lord and Savior Jesus Christ, and suffering because we refuse to obey God's recommendations on how to live successfully while on this earth. The first type of suffering is from obedience and will be rewarded greatly. The second type of suffering is from disobedience which invites death. ("The wages of sin is death," Romans 6:23).

One of the many great things about God is that He allows us to decide how we will live today. No matter what we did yesterday, last month or last year we have another chance today. Will we ignore Him or embrace Him? Will we go our way or His way? Will we choose to live a healthy lifestyle or not?

We need to be forward looking with an occasional backward glance to keep our path straight toward the vision.

If you want to be a little healthier, consider the following:

1) Quiet time: Three parts — Bible Study, prayer, listening (30 minutes a day minimum). If you don't have a spiritual meal at the beginning of your day you will probably be spiritually weak all day. If you don't seek your Heavenly Father, thanking Him for who He is and what He has done; if you don't exercise the power given to you over the enemy; if you don't hold up people and nations and situations in intersession you will probably be spiritually weak all day. If you don't take time to listen for answers and instructions, you will probably be spiritually weak all day. If you don't praise the only One who is worthy, you will probably be spiritually weak all day. As soon as we get busy or when things are going along quite well, many of us give up on our quiet time which is the last thing we should give up.

2) Vision and Purpose: We were created in God's image, therefore, we are creatures capable of vision; we can know where we came from and can "see" where we are going. Man is not only visionary but creative like the Father. We need to be forward looking with purpose with an occasional backward glance to keep our path straight toward the vision. Creative, visionary, purposeful, positive, goal-oriented, hopeful, joyful, peaceful, loving, faithful, persevering, optimistic, courageous, prosperous, and victorious are some of the attributes of Saints. Are you going to heaven? Then you are a Saint. Is your vision a bright and guiding star? Are your goals well established and capable of motivating you? Are these things in agreement with Scriptures? Are you acquainted with God's plan for your life? If the answer to any one of these questions is no, then you have some work to do.

Could you imagine a family who wishes all year for their vacation and when the time comes they jump in the car and drive someplace, any place? Oh, you say, that's ridiculous. How could they prepare if they didn't know where they were going, how long they would be gone, if they were camping or staying in a hotel, etc., etc. Did they take enough money? Did they make arrangements for the dog? Do they need the fishing gear or the ski equipment? I know, it sounds silly, but most of our lives are lived just this way. We are looking forward to heaven (vacation) but we are not properly preparing for it.

The problem with fear is that it paints obstacles bigger than they are.

God doesn't want directionless, improperly prepared people to reign with Him for eternity. He wants Saints! Getting to heaven isn't the end, it's the beginning. We need to use the time we have here to prepare. We need to develop the attributes of Christ since we are going to have the responsibility and authority of rulership.

We have been designed with two halves to our nature, one for working, the other for restoring. Our sympathetic half does our work; our parasympathetic half restores our capacity to work. For example—the downswing does the pendulum's work, the upswing restores the pendulum's capacity to work. This cycling back and forth between working and restoring is needed for success; balance is essential!

When we were born our parasympathetic system came fully developed. That's our restoring half—the one responsible for eating, drinking, sleeping and getting rid of wastes. In contrast, our working half must be developed. As infants we were naturally curious so we explored or worked. Unfortunately, our exploring had its risks and as we grew we gradually found our curiosity replaced by fear.

The problem with fear is that it paints obstacles bigger than they are. So we either withdraw and work too little, or overcompensate and work too much. Withdrawing tilts us toward our parasympathetic side, which tends us toward depression. Overcompensating tilts us toward our sympathetic side, which tends us toward anxiety. Either imbalance makes us feel empty and unfulfilled. Either imbalance interrupts brain chemicals and mechanisms involved in normal motivation and reward.

3) Goal Setting: Goal setting has the opposite effect, while fear causes imbalance, goal setting brings balance. Positive, realistic, obtainable goals promote brain chemicals and mechanisms that enhance this pleasant, rhythmic cooperation between our two systems, and it works automatically.

GOAL SETTING PROCEDURES

1) Write down your goals. They must be realistic and obtainable.
2) Date your goals. Both the date you will start and the date you will achieve your goals.
3) List obstacles to overcome in order to obtain your goals, i.e.: money, time, your personality traits, etc.
4) Identify groups, organizations and individuals you need to work with in order to obtain your goals.
5) List the reasons for obtaining your goals. Why do you want what you want?
6) List the knowledge or information you need in order to obtain your goals.
7) Develop a game plan to obtain your goals. It must be meaningful and specific. What do I have to do or stop doing?
8) Read your goals and plan every morning and every evening, at least twice a day, without fail.
9) DO IT! FOLLOW YOUR PLAN!

WHAT WE EAT IS IMPORTANT, *WHAT WE DON'T EAT* IS IMPORTANT, BUT *HOW* WE EAT IS ALSO VERY IMPORTANT

Perhaps you will need to change your eating habits. Carry the following seven 'tips' with you (possibly make a 3 X 5 card that will fit into your pocket or purse) and read all of the do's and don'ts before every meal and every snack until it becomes a habit.

1) ALWAYS pray before you eat, asking that the food be nourishing to your body. (Does the food you've selected have any nutrients in it?)
2) ALWAYS eat slowly - enjoy it. You will get the same 'full feeling' on 2/3's the amount.
3) ALWAYS chew your food well—digestion begins in your mouth.
4) ALWAYS sit down to eat—so your body can extract the nutrients from the food.
5) NEVER eat when you are upset—the digestive enzymes are not produced properly when upset.
6) NEVER eat "on the run"—digestion is incomplete at best.
7) DON'T drink large amounts just before or during meals as it dilutes the enzymes.

Recently, the pastor at a church we attended announced that he was starting a new teaching series on Wednesday nights. The subject matter would be the book of Daniel. I was very excited because from my own study of the Bible I considered the First Chapter of Daniel to be the most straightforward statement in the whole Bible which says that eating correctly leads to good health while eating incorrectly leads to poor health.

During the last 15 years or so while I've been studying nutrition and the holistic approach to good health, I've always used the Bible as the ultimate standard, the source of truth and proper principles. In all those years, in fact, during my entire church-going life, I have heard thousands of sermons from a variety of Christian pastors, and not one of them focused on good eating habits. It is an extremely rare event when proper eating principles are even mentioned from the pulpit.

Why is this so? As a nutritional counselor, when I studied the Bible looking for answers and advice in my chosen field, I found literally hundreds of passages in Scripture telling of the health promoting aspects of proper eating and proper living. Passages like Leviticus 3:17, "This is a lasting ordinance for the generations to come, wherever you live: you must not eat any fat or any blood." Knowing the adverse effect of fat on things like heart disease, I consider this passage a scriptural principle of healthful eating.

So, on that Wednesday evening I sat in church with high expectations that Daniel's obvious message of good health due to proper eating would at least be mentioned. But, alas, it was not to be. The pastor found a "higher", spiritual meaning in Daniel, Chapter One, that we should not put our love for "things" above our love of God. He didn't mention physical health at all.

While I certainly don't disagree with the Pastor's conclusions, I do believe he missed a wonderful opportunity to help the congregation in a very practical way — better health. I know that this Pastor in particular, and all Christian pastors in general, are very concerned about the health of their congregation because they spend so much time and effort praying for and visiting sick members.

In talking to several members of the clergy, it seems to be a consensus that they pretty much restrict their comments from the pulpit to spiritual matters. Most try to avoid such things as political matters, social issues and other areas such as illness and disease.

This is fully understandable because when God calls a person to become a pastor or an evangelist, that calling is primarily spiritual in nature. There is a burning desire to share the salvation message, the Lordship of Christ, and high moral and spiritual principles of right and wrong. There is also a tremendous pressure on our pastors to always "be right" and "do right". They assume an awesome responsibility of leadership!

The Bible was written for all believers, indeed, for all people, not just for our spiritual leaders. Since your health is your own personal responsibility, NOT your doctor's, NOT your pastor's, NOT your spouse's, it is also your own responsibility to search out the truth. The Bible is true. So study it for all areas of life, including good health.

WORDS TO KNOW

Creative	Visionary	Purposeful
Positive	Goal-Oriented	Hopeful
Joyful	Peaceful	Loving
Faithful	Persevering	Optimistic
Courageous	Prosperous	Victorious

SUMMARY

1. Americans as a whole choose a pretty unhealthy lifestyle.
2. We should start our day with a quiet time, Bible study, prayer, listening.
3. Being positive, forward looking and goal-oriented promote good health.
4. What we eat is important, what we don't eat is important, BUT HOW WE EAT IS VERY IMPORTANT!
5. You are responsible for your own health, NOT your Pastor, NOT your Doctor, NOT your spouse, but YOU.

4

HEALTH PHILOSOPHY HEALTH FRAUD

It will be stated many times in this book that the physical cause of disease is malnutrition and/or poisoning. Some may think that this statement is indefensible because we all *know* that germs cause infectious disease and chemical imbalances cause other diseases. These are undeniable facts **proven** over and over again and taught in every school for a hundred years.

To have any hope of overcoming a lifetime of training, knowing and assuming we must understand the philosophy underlying medical science's approach to healing. This understanding is not at all difficult. It does not require a super intellect or higher education. Using simple logic, common sense and an open mind, it becomes clear.

In simplest terms the philosophy of medical science involves two entities, the disease and the patient. The goal of medicine is to fight the disease and to make the patient better. It's kind of like war; like the 'War on Cancer.' In 1971 we "declared war" on cancer, that heinous disease, that blight on mankind. Killing the disease, however, has become more important than saving the patient. It's exactly like war where casualties are inevitable and the individual is subordinate to the cause of defeating the enemy.

We have all seen those WWII movies where the enemy soldiers occupy a town. The objective of the allied army is to defeat the enemy soldiers and save the

PSALM 1:1

Blessed is the man who does not walk in the counsel of the wicked or stand in the way of sinners or sit in the seat of mockers.

town. The army uses artillery, bombs and bullets to kill the enemy but while trying to liberate the town, they destroy it. That is pretty much what happens in conventional medicine's approach to the cancer patient. The cancer is the enemy attacked with chemotherapy, radiation, surgery, etc. The chemotherapy may kill the cancer but the patient's immune system is weakened and he dies of pneumonia. Or, radiation is applied to throat cancer but the patient can't speak or swallow.

Medical literature often contains statements like, "the procedure was a success but the patient died".

Are these therapies effective? In 1985 the American Cancer Society sponsored cancer research conducted by Robert T. Schimke. Dr. Schimke won the Alfred P. Sloan, Jr. prize for this research. His primary conclusion was that, "chemotherapy tends to make cancer worse."

Look up the word Nosology in a medical dictionary. What do you find? "The science of the classification of diseases." Science must identify and classify things, like kinds of plants or kinds of animals or kinds of diseases. Of course, there are books published that list and classify diseases. It takes almost 100 pages to list all known diseases. The point is, medical science believes that diseases are things, entities. Therefore, you can have a disease, you can get cancer, you can catch a cold; you can give it to someone else. It's a 'thing'. It's somehow separate from the person who has it. That's why medical literature often contains statements like, 'the procedure was a success but the patient died'. In contrast, natural healing, or what we will be referring to as God's way, does not believe that diseases are things.

This difference in philosophy goes back to ancient times. Ironically, Hippocrates, considered to be the "Father of Medicine", believed in natural healing and wrote that food should be our medicine. It was a contemporary of Hippocrates, a philosopher named Democritus, who advocated the opposite view. In 400 BC these two philosophies were called vitalism and atomism, and they are still with us today. Indeed, they have always been with us. Many medical histories have been written. Take a look at *Divided Legacy*, a three volume work by Harris Coulter, if you are interested in the history of medicine.

America's first really famous doctor was a man named Benjamin Rush. He was opinionated and outspoken and did a lot of good things like sign our Declaration of Independence. He believed that the medical doctor should heal the body, not the body heal itself. When asked the question; *Does the body have within itself the ability to heal itself?* Dr. Rush answered, "although a certain power does exist in the organism, it is not strong enough to withstand the onslaughts of disease."

Medical science believes that diseases are caused by either germs or a chemical imbalance.

Medical science believes that diseases are caused by either germs or a chemical imbalance. Germs are microorganisms like viruses, bacteria, fungi, etc. An example of a germ-caused disease would be the flu. Chemical imbalance is when our bodies produce either too little or too much of some active chemical needed for good health. Diabetes would be an example of a disease caused by chemical imbalance, because the body does not make enough insulin. In either case, medicine must intervene by attacking the germs with antibiotics or antiviral drugs, or by supplying deficient, active body chemicals or blocking the production of active body chemicals that are in excess.

On the surface this seems logical, but let's look a little deeper. While it is true that the flu and the flu virus are connected and you can't get the flu without the virus, it is not necessarily true that the virus causes the flu. That's not double talk. In fact, scientific logic confirms it.

Consider the following scenario: 180 people are on board a plane flying non-stop from L.A. to New York. Two of the passengers were just on vacation in Hong Kong where they picked up a flu virus. Because this particular virus is spread through the air and because of an inadequate air filtration system on the aircraft, all the passengers and crew are exposed to the virus. That is, the virus goes inside all the people aboard the plane. Out of the 180 people who received the virus, 16 people get the flu, 164 people don't get the flu. So what do you think? Does the virus cause the flu?

The scientific method of study demands that researchers doing a study use two groups, a control group and an experimental group. The researchers want to find out the difference between the two groups, then look for changes in the experimental group. The researchers create a difference, then look for changes. Whatever the two groups have in common must be automatically eliminated as the cause. Now consider the plane full of people. All the people had the virus so it cannot be the cause. Let's say it another way. If germs caused disease we would all be dead. Every single person in the world is exposed to a large number of germs every single day. Obviously then, germs only contribute to a possible disease situation. The real cause is that our body's own healing powers have been compromised by malnutrition and/or poisoning. The truth is that in a healthy body germs, often cause a strengthening of the body, NOT disease.

Some scientists are now warning us of a disease pandemic unprecedented in the history of mankind.

What has happened over the last sixty years or so? The germ theory has been in vogue. In our exuberance to kill the germs we have created about 100 antibiotics. These antibiotics are dispensed like candy on Halloween. But instead of fewer, weaker germs, we have much stronger germs. In fact, there are now germs that no drug can touch. And how about our body's own healing powers? They have been greatly weakened by these same antibiotics. In fact, some scientists are now warning us of a disease pandemic, unprecedented in the history of mankind.

Chemical Imbalance

Now let's consider the chemical imbalance theory of disease. Basically it says that if the body is not making enough of a needed chemical — supply it artificially in a pill or a shot. If the body is making too much of a chemical, block it's production with a drug. We used diabetes as an example of this type of disease.

The first thing you need to know about any drug therapy is that there are two parts. The first part is the immediate effect of the drug. The second part is the body's reaction or resistance to the drug. Think of it this way. The body has intricate built-in mechanisms for controlling the quantity of all chemicals it makes and needs. The manufacture of these chemicals acts as an automatic inhibitor of further production. It's kind of like a thermostat. You set the thermostat at 75 degrees. As the temperature drops the thermostat turns on the furnace. The furnace produces heat. The heat is noticed by the thermostat and at 75 degrees the furnace is turned off. So, everything is cool, or should I say just right.

In using drug therapy and artificially giving the body a chemical that it should be making itself, the body reacts by making less. Athletes want big, strong muscles for speed and power. Athletes know that testosterone, a male hormone, is necessary to make muscles. Some athletes take artificial testosterones called anabolic steroids. While these athletes grow big, strong muscles, what happens on the inside of their bodies is that their maleness is becoming more feminine for the lack of natural testosterone. If they continue, their livers and kidneys are damaged and many die young.

In the end this type of drug therapy worsens the very disease it is trying to correct. As a person injects artificial insulin to correct a diabetes situation, the body in response makes less insulin. More artificial insulin is then needed to make up the difference.

Drug therapy is based on the belief that the body is better off being controlled from the outside. This belief is understandable when you consider that science also believes that human beings evolved from lower organisms, that evolution is still going on and that science might control or at least influence future evolution. Such a belief system would have no compunction in wrestling control away from our body's innate intelligence. As a Christian, believing in creation, I find any notion that denies the existence of God to be offensive, and of course, incorrect.

Iatrogenic Disease

Do you know what the word iatrogenic means? Genic means the start, or origin or cause. Iatros is the Greek word for doctor or physician. So iatrogenic means doctor caused. According to a report in the Journal of the American Medical Association, 2 1/2% of ICU patients died of iatrogenic disease. About 35% of patients at a university hospital had iatrogenic diseases according to the New England Journal of Medicine. It is estimated that about 700,000 people die every year due to iatrogenic disease.

There are two types of iatrogenic disease, avoidable and unavoidable. Avoidable iatrogenic illness comes as a result of doctors' errors. Anyone can make a mistake, even doctors. Unavoidable iatrogenic disease is from the effects of drugs and other treatments. Avoidable iatrogenic disease is the reason malpractice insurance is so high, but the overwhelming majority of iatrogenic disease is unavoidable. It is simply part of the system. It is unavoidable because the underlying philosophy, the underlying belief system, is incorrect, or at least subordinate to a higher principle.

How can this be? After all, the FDA demands that a drug be proven safe and effective before it can be used. In fact, it costs about 70 million dollars to develop and test a new drug. Extremely elaborate and carefully designed scientific double blind studies are run and rerun. Every effort is taken to properly match the control and experimental groups to eliminate every possible variable except the drug being tested and the placebo given. And yet, in a high percentage of cases, after actual experience in the 'real world' a drug is found to be ineffective or unsafe and removed from the market. The diet drugs Phen Fen are a recent example.

Could one reason be the very nature of the tests? These scientific double blind studies demand that the patient be totally ignorant of what he is receiving and have absolutely no control over the proceedings. Could these double blind studies provoke a feeling of helplessness in the patient, and could this helplessness itself be a factor in the test?

Norman Cousins is the author of a book called *The Healing Heart.* In this book Mr. Cousins wrote about how he recovered from a very serious heart attack. He used some unconventional therapies like humor. He asked his friends to tell him jokes. He made his surroundings very pleasant, bright cheerful rooms, soft easy music, etc. He began exercising and walked several miles each day. Everything appeared to be going well — he felt good — he was recovering nicely. At one point his doctor asked him to come in for a stress test. Mr. Cousins did so. At the end of the test his doctor wanted to admit him to the hospital for emergency heart surgery, the test results were that bad. Mr. Cousins refused. He knew he was getting better. He was able to exercise every day. He felt good and strong.

One of the great things about truth is that it is self sustaining.

Mr. Cousins went home and considered the matter for a couple of days. He then called his doctor and asked if he could take the stress test again. His doctor agreed. But this time instead of taking the test in the cold, drab clinic, Mr. Cousins asked if he could take the test in his own bright, cheerful room. And he asked if he could control the test, that is, the speed and elevation of the treadmill. Again his doctor agreed. He passed the second stress test with flying colors! He didn't need heart surgery! Can our surroundings, our environment and a feeling of helplessness effect our physiology to such a degree? I believe they can and do.

One of the great things about truth is that it is self sustaining. We don't have to spend a lot of time, effort or energy to support the truth because the truth ultimately supports itself. In science we call these truths laws, like the law of gravity. One of the most fundamental laws in science is the Second Law of

Thermodynamics. This law has to do with the flow of energy. This law states—*NATURAL PROCESSES MOVE FROM ORDER TO DISORDER.* The Second Law of Thermodynamics does not rule out the possibility of creating order out of disorder, it merely states that such a reversal of the natural flow requires an influx of energy, and all systems consume more energy than they produce. In other words—there is no perpetual motion machine.

The Second Law of Thermodynamics is why you can burn paper into smoke, ash and heat, but you can't unburn smoke, ash and heat to make paper. It is the reason that if you placed a bowling ball on a sloped roof it would roll down. You could keep the bowling ball on the roof but it would take a lot of energy to do so. Think of this silly analogy ... let's say you bought 100 ping pong balls and numbered them from 1 to 100 and put them all in a box. It would take you a certain amount of energy to take them out of the box and line them up on a table. It would take more energy to line them up in numerical order. That's the Second Law of Thermodynamics.

Energy can be heat, motion (work), light, information, or other forms. Our human bodies have within them intelligence, or information energy that enables them to grow and repair. You could call it natural healing power. I will simply call it life. As soon as this intelligence, this information, this energy, this life leaves the body, the body begins to go from order to disorder. The body begins to decay.

The thing that either supports or erodes our life force energy is the environment we put it in. There are really two environments, an internal environment which the body should control and an external environment which we should control. Trying to override the body's control of our internal environment is like trying to repair a cadaver. We don't have the information or energy to do it. And while there is life left in a body, the body will always resist our efforts to do so.

Gen. 2:7—"*The Lord God formed the man from the dust of the ground and breathed into his nostrils the breath of life, and man became a living being.*"

HEALTH FRAUD

For many years and with great success the medical establishment has been trying to establish and enforce laws against **health fraud**. Of course, we are all against fraud (untruth) of all kinds. Part of the problem is the way the establishment defines **health fraud**. The Deputy Commissioner of the FDA, John Norris, defined it as anything done by anyone who is not a licensed medical doctor. That means that anyone who chooses anything other than approved medical therapy is a victim of **health fraud**.

Drugs only have effects, NOT side effects.

The Professional's Guide to Health & Nutrition Fraud, says that most victims are "alienated, desperate, unsuspecting, gullible people." Studies show, however, that the more education a person has, the more likely they will seek alternative therapies, including natural healing therapies. Many times these alternative therapies seek to build up a person's general state of health rather than using specific drugs for specific diseases. The California Medical Association warns against such practices in their publication The Professional's Guide to Health & Nutrition Fraud, "be wary of claims that a product may be used for multiple health problems. Generally speaking, such products exist only in the portfolios of con artists."

William T. Jarvis, president of the National Council Against Health Fraud stated that there are many persons practicing health fraud, people like "alchemists, witches, herbalists, health food therapists and faith healers." According to Mr. Jarvis then, many Christian pastors are practicing health fraud. Does the Bible address this issue? James 5:14-16 (NIV), "Is any of you sick? He should call the elders of the church to pray over him and anoint him with oil in the name of the Lord. And the prayer offered in faith will make the sick person well; the Lord will raise him up. If he has sinned, he will be forgiven. Therefore confess your sins to each other and pray for each other so that you may be healed. The prayer of a righteous man is powerful and effective." In 1 Corinthians 12:9, Paul tells us that God gave many gifts to mankind, including the "gifts of healing." Of course, there are scores of accounts where Jesus himself healed hundreds of people.

Mr. Jarvis and Mr. Norris and many others within the established medical community would have us believe that drug therapy is the only legitimate path to healing, that everything else is fraudulent. Medicine is NOT the *only* path to health. It is NOT the *best* path to health. It is NOT even the *preferred* path to health. Medicine's attempt to legislate away all competition is doomed to failure because the truth is, and the truth supports itself.

One final thought before we move on. Why don't you prayerfully read and consider Revelation, Chapter 18. In the last part of verse 23 it says, "By your magic spell (sorcery) all the nations were led astray." The Greek word John used that is translated magic spell or sorcery was Pharmakia. That's the root word that pharmacy and pharmaceuticals come from. Pharmakia simply means drugs. Could it be that in the last days all the world will be led astray by drugs? Study Revelation Chapter 18 and decide for yourself.

THE PHILOSOPHY OF REGENERATION

Unfortunately, regeneration is not the prevailing philosophy in Western society! We have been taught all our lives that the body is a machine and when something goes wrong we have to have it fixed. This is the philosophy of substitution.

Substitution may not necessarily be incorrect, however, it is definitely subordinate to regeneration. To say it another way, substitution may be appropriate during crisis situations for short periods of time, but is not appropriate for non-critical situations or for long periods of time.

Regeneration is*—allowing, wholeness, balance, and harmony*

Substitution is*—forcing, isolates, intervention, and upsetting*

Let's take a look at what some "reformed" medical doctors have to say on this very subject.

Robert D. Willix, Jr., M.D. from his book *You Can Feel Good All the Time*

"I'm a medical doctor and I used to look at things the same way as the medical establishment. Basically, their view is that the body is a sort of machine you fix when it breaks down. I shucked off this dangerous, mistaken point of view and learned how human beings really work.

Over the past 40 years, evidence has been piling up that the way the body works is totally different from what the medical profession thinks.

Thousands of other doctors all over the United States are doing the same thing I'm doing. We are painfully "unlearning" all the myths we used to believe. The old way of looking at things is under assault. The walls are crumbling."

Robert S. Mendelsohn, M.D. from his book *How To Raise a Healthy Child in Spite of Your Doctor*

"This book reflects my belief that in pediatrics, as in other specialties, a great deal of bad medicine is practiced in the United States. That does not imply, however, that doctors have less integrity or compassion than the rest of mankind. The shortcomings lie within the philosophy and teaching of medicine, not in the character of those who are taught.

Doctors aren't culprits. Like their patients, they are victims of the system. They are the first to be impaired by medical education's preoccupation with intervention rather than prevention, its infatuation with drugs and technology, and the indefensible rituals, mores and egotistical attitudes that are burned into the brain of

Doctors aren't culprits. Like their patients, they are victims of the system.

every student who survives the rigid and often irrelevant curriculum and training. They emerge with their heads so stuffed with institutionalized foolishness that there is no room left for common sense.

I don't exempt myself from this criticism of other pediatricians. I confess that I began my medical practice believing most of what I had been taught, and my patients paid the price for many years. Fortunately, perhaps because I began teaching medical students myself, I learned to question many of the medical principles that had been drilled into me and to suspect every new drug, surgical procedure, and medical "innovation" that came along. I soon discovered that most of them couldn't withstand rigorous scientific evaluation and that an incredible percentage of the "wonder drugs" and "revolutionary procedures" soon disappeared when it was discovered that they did more harm than good."

The Bible is actually relevant as an instruction manual for our day-to-day life.

Eugene D. Robin, M.S., professor of medicine and physiology at Stanford Medical School in his book *Matters of Life and Death: Risks Vs. Benefits of Medical Care.*

"There are serious flaws in the basic processes by which diagnostic and therapeutic measures are introduced and used in medicine. You will be advised to consult doctors only when you believe that you are truly ill. By restricting your medical encounters to those that are absolutely necessary you will be avoiding the risks inherent in most diagnostic and therapeutic procedures. Even a decision to consult a doctor is a serious and potentially risky one."

Dr. Linus Pauling, Two time Nobel Laureate and famous scientist and activist in his book *How to Live Longer and Feel Better*

"I believe that in general the treatment of disease by the use of substances, such as ascorbic acid, that are normally present in the human body and are required for life is to be preferred to treatment by the use of powerful synthetic substances or plant products, which may, and usually do, have undesirable side effects. I have coined the term orthomolecular medicine for the preservation of good health and the treatment of disease by varying the concentrations in the human body of substances that are normally present in the body and are required for health. Dr. Bernard Rimland has emphasized my point by suggesting that conventional medicine, which uses drugs, be called toximolecular medicine."

These are not isolated incidents of crackpot doctors that have a cross to bear against the medical establishment. They are a few examples of hundreds of long term, well respected doctors and scientists who have come to the conclusion that the most basic underlying principles of western medicine are subordinate to higher principles. In other words, the philosophy of substitution is dangerous and subordinate to the philosophy of regeneration! After all, when you plant an acorn you don't expect a rose to grow. The information in the acorn can only produce an oak tree, but it knows how to grow that oak tree perfectly!

I believe that the Bible is actually relevant as an instruction manual for our day-to-day life and I just can't resist one more guidance from Scripture to conclude this chapter.

Colossians 2:3-4 (NIV),—"*Christ, in whom are hidden all treasures of wisdom and knowledge. I tell you this so that no one may deceive you by fine-sounding arguments.*

(Verse 8) *See to it that no one takes you captive through hollow and deceptive philosophy, which depends on human tradition and the basic principles of this world rather than on Christ.* (Verse 23) *Such regulations indeed have an appearance of wisdom, with... their harsh treatment of the body, but they lack any value in restraining sensual indulgence.*"

WORDS TO KNOW

Nosology	Chemical Imbalance	Pharmakia
Vitalism	Anabolic Steroids	Atomism
Iatrogenic	Antibiotics	Placebo

The Second Law of Thermodynamics

SUMMARY

1. The physical cause of most disease is either malnutrition or poisoning or both.
2. We have been taught all of our lives that germs or chemical imbalances cause disease.
3. Medical science thinks that diseases are things—are entities.
4. Medical science tries to kill the disease.
5. Chemotherapy tends to make cancer worse.
6. Natural healing does not think diseases are things, instead it feeds and strengthens the patient.
7. Science believes and teaches evolution.
8. Most iatrogenic diseases are unavoidable.
9. Medical testing leaves the patient with a feeling of helplessness.
10. The establishment claims that anything outside of established medical practice is **health fraud**—people like alchemists, witches, herbalists, health food therapists and faith healers.
11. Many doctors are rejecting the establishment's claims and are embracing natural healing principles.

5

THE EVILS OF THIS WORLD

Many people will debate the points in this book. They will say that we live in an age of reason. They believe that mankind is becoming ever more enlightened. They will argue that the government is here for our protection, that everything is getting better, that we are headed in the right direction. Well, everyone is entitled to their own opinion, but opinions change as the truth becomes known.

1 TIMOTHY 4:1

The Spirit clearly says that in later times some will abandon the faith and follow deceiving spirits and things taught by demons.

Let's look at some of examples of unreasonable, unenlightened and non-protective things that are going on.

Fluorine, the most corrosive element in all of nature and one of the worst poisons; is deliberately added to our water supply, is added to products like toothpaste and mouthwash and floss, and even put in our baby vitamins. (See Chapter 9).

Aspartame, an artificial sweetener that breaks down into a deadly neurotoxin, is added to thousands of our processed food products. (See Chapter 10).

One of the most heinous events imaginable is being practiced in the United States of America. It's called partial birth abortion. In this procedure, as a baby is being born but just as its head comes out of the womb a so-called "doctor" pushes an instrument through its soft skull and sucks out part of the brain. (As this book is being written Congress is trying to muster enough votes to override a presidential veto of a bill prohibiting this practice).

Let's turn our attention to a few recent court decisions:

Harvey Vs. Cobb County, 1993. Even though the Ten Commandments are engraved in stone in the U.S. Supreme Court, and despite the fact that they make up the basis of civil law, they may NOT be displayed at any public courthouse.

It is unconstitutional for students to see the Ten Commandments because they might read them or respect them or obey them.

Lanner Vs. Wimmer, 1981 - Stone Vs. Graham, 1980 - Ring Vs. Grand Forks Public School District, 1980. These court decisions stated that it was unconstitutional for students to see the Ten Commandments because they might read them or respect them or obey them.

Wallace Vs. Jaffree 1985. Even when the wording of a bill is constitutionally acceptable, it becomes unconstitutional if the law maker who wrote it had a religious activity in mind.

Roberts Vs. Madigan, 1990. It is unconstitutional for a teacher to be seen with a Bible at school or for a classroom library to include books dealing with Christianity.

Warsaw Vs. Tehachapi, 1990. It is unconstitutional for a public cemetery to have a planter shaped like a cross because someone might look at that cross and suffer "emotional distress" which would be an injury-in-fact.

Stein Vs. Oshinsky, 1965 - Collins Vs. Chandler Unified School District, 1981 - Bishop Vs. Aronov, 1991 - Duran Vs. Nitsche, 1991. The freedom of speech and freedom of the press are guaranteed to both teachers and students unless the topic is religious, then the speech or press becomes unconstitutional.

During the course of our study on health and how to eat and live, you are going to read and hear many things that will be new, and even some things that will contradict what you have learned all your life. Since what you choose to believe will have an enormous effect on what you will receive from this book, we will be looking at the base causes for the evils of this world and why things have become so distorted.

What is it about the human experience that leads to anything other than total loveliness, peacefulness and joyfulness? In the aggregate, it is man's rebellion against God. Some of us are bold enough to call it sin, while most of us would prefer a watered down, white-washed, less critical notion. But let's be bold. Where did sin come from and how did it originate? The possibility of sin came from man's free moral agency, his freedom of choice. But it originated in the heart and mind of the person we call Satan, in the place we now call the Garden of Eden.

Satan helped produce that first sin and every one since. And when sin came into the world so did sickness and disease and misery of every kind. Therefore, as a part of our study of health, we should review who this guy Satan is, what he wants to do, and how to spoil his plan.

Satan has had a long and colorful history. God created him perfect and beautiful and powerful and a lot of other wonderful things, and called his name Lucifer. But pride got to him and he rebelled against God, and tried to make himself equal to or higher than God. So God cast him down to the earth. Have you ever wondered why God cast him to the earth rather than some barren planet in an unknown galaxy on the other side of the universe? Or why God created man and placed him on the earth? Do you think that God forgot Satan was here? Probably not! These thoughts bring up lots of other questions which are outside the realm of our present endeavor. Suffice it to say that God must have had His reasons.

So mankind and Satan (along with his fallen angels and demons) have been sharing this world for the last 6,000 years or so. Of course, men come and go, (they die) but Satan came and stayed. He was not only created with incredible intelligence but he has had plenty of time to perfect his skills. Needless to say, the devil is a formidable opponent for man, but fortunately, not for God.

Let's take a quick look at what the Scriptures tell us about Satan; not to lift him up, but to recognize his schemes and to be able to use the same power that raised Christ from the dead to resist and defeat him.

The Bible tells us ever so plainly why the world is full of deceit and hatred and sickness and misery of every sort. Satan is the ruler of this world. Revelation 12:12 tells us, "But woe to the earth and the sea, because the devil has gone down to you! He is filled with fury, because he knows that his time is short." Thank God for His grace that as believers we don't have to be of this world and under Satan's control. Ephesians 2:1-2 says, "As for you, you were dead in your transgressions and sins, in which you used to live when you followed the ways of this world and of the ruler of the kingdom of the air, the spirit who is now at work in those who are disobedient." John agrees with Paul in I John 5:19, "We know that we are children of God, and that the whole world is under the control of the evil one." Yes, Satan is the god of this world during this present age and has some control over unbelievers. II Corinthians 4:4 says, "The god of this age has blinded the minds of unbelievers, ..."

The devil is not omnipresent but he has plenty of help; there are the fallen angels and also the demons that he commands. Just because we are believers doesn't mean that we are safe. Satan is always fighting against the Saints. I Thessalonians 2:18 gives us a good example, "For we wanted to come to you—certainly I, Paul, did, again and again—but Satan stopped us." Paul makes it clear that there is a war going on. In Ephesians 6:12 he tells us, "for our struggle is not against flesh and blood, but against the rulers, against the authorities, against the powers of this dark world and against the spiritual forces of evil in the heavenly realms." Study the 10th chapter of Daniel to catch a glimpse of this warfare. Daniel 10:20, "Soon I will return to fight against the prince of Persia, and when I go, the prince of Greece will come." David also came under attack. In I Chronicles 21:1 it says, "Satan rose up against Israel and incited David to take a census of Israel." Satan is at war with the Saints great and small; David, Daniel, Paul. Do you think somehow you are exempt?

There are no conscientious objectors in the army of the Saints. You either recognize the situation, put on God's armor and use His weapons; or you get beat up! Satan is not a nice guy. He is NOT fair! He won't leave you alone even if you leave him alone.

- The devil is a tempter. Matthew 4:3, Mark 1:13, I Corinthians 7:5, Genesis 3:1, I Thessalonians 3:5
- The devil will always try to get to you again and again. Luke 4:13
- The devil steals God's Word from our hearts. Luke 8:12, Mark 4:15
- The devil is a murderer. John 8:44
- The devil is a liar, and the father of lies. John 8:44, Revelation 2:24, Genesis 3:4
- Unbelievers are under the power of the devil. Acts 10:38, Revelation 2:9, 13; 3:9
- The devil is the "father" of the unbeliever. Acts 13:10, I John 3:10
- We must never give the devil a foothold in our lives. Ephesians 4:27, I Timothy 5:15
- The believer must fight against the devil's schemes. Ephesians 6:11, II Corinthians 2:11
- The devil traps us. I Timothy 3:7, II Timothy 2:26
- The devil enslaves us. II Timothy 2:26, Luke 13:16
- The devil holds the power of death. Hebrews 2:14
- The devil wants to devour you. I Peter 5:8

- The devil is a sinner from the beginning. I John 3:8
- The devil puts us in prison. Revelation 2:10
- The devil leads the whole world astray. Revelation 12:9
- Satan puts thoughts in our mind. I Chronicles 21:1, Matthew 16:23, Mark 8:33
- Satan accuses the believers. Job 1:9-11; 2:4-5, Psalm 109:6, Zechariah 3:1, Revelation 12:10
- Satan attacks our health. Job 2:7, II Corinthians 12:7
- Satan can control people. Luke 22:3, John 13:27, Acts 5:3
- Satan asks God for permission to attack us. Luke 22:31
- Men get turned over to Satan. I Corinthians 5:5, I Timothy 1:20
- Satan can seem beautiful. II Corinthians 11:14
- Satan is always fighting against the Saints. I Thessalonians 2:18
- Satan deceives all mankind. II Thessalonians 2:9
- Satan is the ruler of this world. John 12:31, 14:30, 16:11, Ephesians 2:2, Matthew 4:8-9, I John 5:19
- Satan is the god of this age. II Corinthians 4:4

This is certainly not a complete list. I urge you to continue this study on your own.

I Corinthians 3:16 says, "Don't you know that you yourselves are God's temple and that God's Spirit lives in you?" The Almighty God of the universe lives in every believer in the form of the Holy Spirit. When a person can by faith apprehend that truth, he gains great authority. But Satan lies to us and hides that truth from us. You see, Satan is a liar and the father of lies. He has had 6,000 years to perfect his schemes, and on top of that he was created one of the most intelligent and powerful beings ever. He stands against God and God's purpose.

Satan's lies can be so complete as to be a fact. A fact is something that is indisputable using our mind and our five senses. But never the less, a fact can be a lie from Satan. Satan is the god of this world. Satan is the ruler of this age. He has legal authority and control over this world at this time. God, of course, is not of this world and neither are we (believers). God's kingdom is eternal and infinite, while this world is corporal and finite. This world will pass away, GOD'S WORD WON'T! God's kingdom is reality, this world is but shadow. What the carnal mind considers to be a fact, can be a lie. Whatever stands against God's Word is a lie whether it is a fact or not, i.e.: The Bible says, "… and by His wounds we are healed. Isaiah 53:5.

Most believers agree in principle with the Scriptures quoted and the arguments presented, but quickly fall away when putting them into practice.

Believers are not of this world. We are called to separate ourselves from this world. We are merely sojourners in this world. It is only when we care about the things of this world that it has any power over us. As soon as we apprehend God's truth, by faith, Satan's lie disappears. We will receive the healing here and now that we have in heavenly places. We will receive right here and now that peace and joy that we have in heavenly places.

God's Word is true here and now and anywhere and anytime. Anything that is not perfectly within God's Word is a lie, is not real, is an illusion. Oh, the misery that we allow Satan to heap upon us simply because we refuse to believe God's Word rather than our senses.

God, in His mighty provision, has given us everything we need to become overcomers. I John 5:4-5 says, "for everyone born of God overcomes the world. This is the victory that has overcome the world, even our faith. Who is it that overcomes the world? Only he who believes that Jesus is the Son of God." Resist the devil and he will flee from you (James 4:7). God put

Satan under believers' feet (Romans 16:20).

When God created Adam and Eve, He gave them dominion over the earth—that is, a legal title deed to the earth. (Gen. 1:26). When Adam and Eve sinned, they lost their legal ownership of the world and Satan claimed it for himself.

Apparently, the only legal way for the undisputed rights to the earth (title deed) to be reinstated to God and mankind was for a perfectly sin-free and righteous man to pay the penalty for sin, laid down by God in Gen. 3:3, which is death. Knowing this, God sent His son to be born of a virgin. Jesus was a real man. He faced every temptation of Satan and the world. Yet He remained absolutely righteous in every thought, every emotion, every word and every deed. Jesus, a totally righteous man, then gave up His life to pay the price for every sin ever committed and to regain the legal rights to the world. He also overcame the devil and death and He set mankind free.

Anyone who simply believes that Jesus Christ is the Son of God, died for the sins of the world and rose from the dead in victory, is credited with the righteousness of Christ and receives a home in heaven forever. Every believer in Jesus also receives the authority to use the very same power that raised Christ from the dead, to resist Satan, all temptations of the world and our old human nature, and to follow God's commandments, rules and suggestions of how to live while we are in this world.

The only power that Satan now has over any believer in Christ is the power that the believer gives to Satan by his ignorance or his apathy or his disobedience. Through faith and prayer believers have awesome power! Power to overcome the devil and the evils of this world in their life.

Most believers agree in principle with the Scriptures quoted and the arguments presented, but quickly fall away when putting them into practice. I've heard many Christians say "that couldn't happen in the United States" or "that's too rotten, the government wouldn't allow that". Sugar is a good example. The government says it promotes cavities but otherwise is a perfectly good "food". It's not a food but an insidious drug. Oh, sure it gives some temporary carnal pleasure but in the long run is responsible for untold misery. Many, many products and practices that are a common and integral part of the world system are really the brainchild of the devil. He is slick. He deceives and corrupts incessantly.

But Satan and his world system are only part of the problem. Every human was born with a sinful, carnal nature. Paul writes about himself and all of humanity in Romans 7:18, "I know that nothing good lives in me, that is, in my sinful nature." Jeremiah 17:9 says, "The heart is deceitful above all things...". "By appealing to the lustful desires of sinful human nature, they entice people" (II Peter 2:18). And again Paul writes about the unbeliever in Ephesians 4;19, "Having lost all sensitivity, they have given themselves over to sensuality so as to indulge in every kind of impurity, with a continual lust for more."

Perhaps that is why the Psalmist warns us in Psalm 1:1, "Blessed is the man who does not walk in the counsel of the wicked, or stand in the way of sinners or sit in the seat of mockers." To me this simply means not to seek the advise of the ungodly or accept the "wisdom" of the world. James tells us in James 3:15-16, "such 'wisdom' does not come down from heaven but is earthly, unspiritual, of the devil. For where you have envy and selfish ambition, there you find disorder and every evil practice." Investigate and see if the motive (of most things of the world) isn't selfish ambition. Paul agreed when he wrote to Timothy in II Timothy 4:3-4, "For the time will come when men will not put up with sound doctrine. Instead, to suit their own desires, they will gather around them a great number of teachers to say what their itching ears want to hear. They will turn their ears away from the truth and turn aside to myths."

These passages apply equally well to our physical

being as our spiritual being, but most Christians only consider them for the latter. It's a shame too, because believers have every right to be physically, mentally and spiritually vital and healthy.

So, as always, its up to you to choose. You can believe that there is no devil or that he has no power, and do nothing about him; or you can learn his ways and take the appropriate steps to neutralize him. You can believe that human nature is basically good and loving, or you can believe the Bible and crucify the flesh daily. You can have faith in the world's methods and traditions and believe that things are getting better or you can put your trust in the unseen kingdom that will last forever.

I Corinthians 2:12-14 - "We have not received the spirit of the world but the Spirit who is from God that we may understand what God has freely given us. This is what we speak, not in words taught us by human wisdom but in words taught by the Spirit, expressing spiritual truths in spiritual words. The man without the Spirit does not accept the things that come from the Spirit of God, for they are foolishness to him, and he cannot understand them, because they are spiritually discerned".

So, when you hear or read something new or something that contradicts what you have thought for years, or something that sounds radical, please consider it thoughtfully and prayerfully, compare it to the principles laid down in God's Word, then decide. But whatever you have faith in, whatever you believe, act on it! Because as James tells us, faith without works is dead. (James 2:20). Knowledge is useless until it is put into action. Start judging yourself on your actions instead of on your intentions and you will make the most of the knowledge you receive. It's simple but it is not easy.

One final Scripture verse for those who still believe that the world system is okay. James 4:4, "You adulterous people, don't you know that friendship with the world is hatred toward God? Anyone who chooses to be a friend of the world becomes an enemy of God."

WORDS TO KNOW

Unconstitutional

Omnipresent

SUMMARY

1. There are a great number of products and events that seem to be okay or even good, that are really very bad for us.
2. The world is NOT becoming more civilized, more enlightened or better.
3. Satan is the god of this world at this time.
4. God's word is absolute truth.
5. Believers have everything they need to become overcomers.

MARK THIS DOWN!

If you decide to honor God with your eating habits—you will get resistance from the enemy!

6

CARDIOVASCULAR DISEASE

PROVERBS 16:22

Understanding is a fountain of Life to those who have it, but folly brings punishment to fools.

Cardiovascular disease is still the number one killer in the U.S., accounting for nearly half of all deaths. About one out of three deaths in the U.S. is caused by heart attacks alone. The rest is from stroke, hypertension and other blood vessel problems. The amazing fact is that the heart attack was completely unknown until early in this century. The first clinical description of coronary thrombosis (heart attack) was made in 1912. The world famous heart specialist, Dr. Paul Dudley White who treated President Eisenhower for his heart attack in the early 1950's, did not see his first case of myocardial infarction until 1921. Hard to believe? Yes, but it is true. The coronary heart attack, which is almost exclusively the end result of atherosclerosis of the coronary arteries, was completely unknown until early in this century. That means, of course, that the U.S. is in the midst of an unprecedented disease epidemic of modern origin.

What is a heart attack anyway? And what causes one? Most people have a pretty good idea. But maybe we should go over it. A myocardial infarction, or in common language, a heart attack, occurs when a portion of the heart muscle dies. Part of the heart dies when the blood supply is cut off. This is caused by coronary thrombosis, or a blood clot forming in the artery, stopping the blood flow. So, myocardial infarction, coronary thrombosis and heart attack are used synonymously. The blood clot is either caused by platelets sticking together or a chunk of plaque breaking loose in an atheromatous plaque buildup on the inside of the arteries. Therefore, a heart attack is the end result of a more general disease process in which fatty deposits are laid down in the arteries. This disease is known as atherosclerosis. There is another term we need to explain - angina pectoris. This is a syndrome of intermittent chest pains usually precipitated by exercise, or emotional stress. While angina pectoris is not a heart attack, it is prima-facie evidence of coronary insufficiency caused by atherosclerosis. There are a number of other problems caused by atherosclerosis. Chief among these are:

The heart attack was completely unknown until early in this century.

1) Strokes
2) Hypertension
3) Peripheral arterial disease like gangrene
4) Aneurysms
5) Senility
6) Male Sexual Impotency
7) Dizziness
8) Transient paralyses
9) Forgetfulness
10) Loss of mental alertness

Of course, this brings up another question; what causes atherosclerosis? That question was answered in Chapter One, but, according to the American Heart Association, the culprit is "Serum Cholesterol". Cholesterol, a fatty substance found normally in all living tissue, is essential to health. However, when there is too much cholesterol in the blood, it can build up on the walls of the arteries, narrow their passageways, and set the stage for heart attack and stroke. A physician can measure the amount of cholesterol in the blood, and prescribe drug and diet regimens to maintain it within a normal range. Well, there you have it. Cholesterol is the villain! The cholesterol theory has become so thoroughly accepted as God-given truth that most authorities explain away in a most illogical manner any evidence which would cast a shadow of a doubt on its unquestionable validity. If you go along with the cholesterol theory, here is what they say you should do about it:

- Avoid foods that contain large amounts of saturated fats.
- Completely eliminate the foods that contain too much cholesterol (organ meats, egg yolks, shrimp, etc.).
- Eliminate butter, cream, pastries, fried foods, etc.
- Use polyunsaturated oils.
- Use fish, chicken and turkey instead of red meat.
- Eat broiled foods instead of fried foods.
- Use skim milk when making desserts such as chocolate pudding (don't you love that one?).
- See your doctor for a cholesterol check and cholesterol lowering drugs when necessary.

Let's say that you agree with the cholesterol theory and get your serum cholesterol level checked. For those people a discussion of the cholesterol numbers is in order. Notice numbers (plural), because simply knowing your total cholesterol will not give you the whole story. Let's first consider total cholesterol. An infant is born with a total cholesterol level of about 70, but it goes up to about 150 in the first couple of years. It stabilizes at about that level until the late teens, then starts going up again, to an average of about 220 which is the median level of adults in the United States, Canada and similar cultures.

Until recently, most doctors did not consider cholesterol levels excessive until they got over 300. Even the cardiology textbooks of the very recent past say not to worry unless a person's total cholesterol exceeds 250. This is very hard to understand because we have known for years that the average first time heart attack victim had a total cholesterol level of 240.

But total cholesterol is only part of the story. We also must consider the kinds of cholesterol—or more accurately, the ways cholesterol is moved around inside the body. Cholesterol does not travel in the body all by itself. It must be carried by something. That something is little fatty substances called lipoproteins. There are five kinds of lipoproteins, four of which have a tendency to allow cholesterol to accumulate inside our arteries. So we will group these four together and call them low-density lipoprotein, or LDL. Therefore, LDL carried cholesterol is bad because it has a tendency to collect in our blood vessels and become atherosclerosis. The bad news is that for most Americans the great majority of cholesterol is carried by LDL. Fortunately, there is a fifth lipoprotein that turns out to be good. This is called high-density lipoprotein or HDL. HDL apparently picks up cholesterol from deposits all over the body and takes it to the liver where it is made into bile, a digestive enzyme that breaks down fat in our digestive track.

Okay, we know that there is more to cholesterol than just the total cholesterol number, and, medical wisdom is now saying that anything over 200 in total cholesterol is considered dangerously high. So, here is how the LDL-HDL fit in. Recent research indicates that high LDL and low HDL puts a person at high risk to have a heart attack. This research also suggests that the ratio between total cholesterol and HDL is important. For example, if your total cholesterol is 200 and HDL is 50, your ratio is 4 which is considered very good. But if your total cholesterol is 210 and your HDL is 30, your ratio is 7, which is very bad. Apparently the optimal ratio is 3.5, but anything under 4.5 is considered good.

So here is the current advise from our medical friends. If your total cholesterol is over 200 you are at high risk. If LDL is over 160 you are at high risk. If your total cholesterol/HDL ratio is over 4.5 you are at high risk. If you fall into any or all of these high risk areas, you should comply with the diet and drug suggestions enumerated earlier, according to the medical establishment. And that is probably pretty good advice because there has definitely been established a correlation between these levels of blood cholesterol and the probability of having a heart attack.

However, the establishment is overlooking some vital information in that they have failed to prove a causative relationship between cholesterol and heart attack. Let's use an example to illustrate this point. Supose that a man gets drunk every Friday night. If that is all the information we have we might conclude that Friday's cause the man to drink. If we add a fact that he gets paid on Fridays, we might change our minds. It has been known for decades that atheromatous plaques are composed mainly of cholesterol, therefore, we blame cholesterol for atherosclerosis. This conclusion ignores other vital information. Cholesterol has been made the villain of heart disease while polyunsaturated fats have been pushed on the consumer as a solution. Both of these ideas will be found incorrect.

Cholesterol is not the enemy that everyone would have us believe.

Cholesterol is not the enemy that everyone would have us believe. It is essential to many body functions. Cholesterol works together with other lipids in the body to maintain a harmonious system. The liver uses cholesterol to produce bile salts for proper fat digestion and absorption by the body. Cholesterol is important to the hormonal system, as a precursor in making vitamin D, and as a conductor for nerve impulses. Most importantly, cholesterol works to build and maintain the cell membrane. Cholesterol and other lipids are central to the structure of every cell in the body, and are a controlling factor in the ability of the cell to absorb nutrients. Cholesterol isn't some hideous poison lurking in our food to kill us. As a matter of fact, cholesterol is made by our own bodies. It has been shown repeatedly that the less cholesterol ingested from dietary sources, the more the body must make for its own use. In fact, if you avoid cholesterol altogether, your body may actually produce more cholesterol than normal. Furthermore, studies show that those people who have been following the low cholesterol diet to an extreme degree, prove to be victims of tumors and are saddled with premature aging and tissue breakdown.

We have already established the heart attack as a modern day killer. If cholesterol was the main cause, this could not be so because cholesterol has been around as long as mankind. Therefore, saturated fat and too much cholesterol are erroneously blamed. The truth is that there are many large populations of people who eat large amounts of saturated fat and lots of cholesterol and do not have any heart attacks. There are tribes in Africa that live primarily on a meat and milk diet, generation after generation, with no heart attacks. The dietary fat intake of the Eskimos is simply hard to believe — an adult may eat several pounds of blubber (about as saturated a fat as exists) at one sitting. This fantastic dietary pattern is followed for a lifetime, without producing heart attacks or strokes. Given these examples, along with the fact that our bodies can produce 3000 to 4000 milligrams of cholesterol every day casts serious doubts on the theory that excess cholesterol causes heart attacks. There is a correlation, that's obvious, but not a causative relationship.

All of the talk about the cholesterol numbers presupposes that the tests are accurate. But, the test for serum cholesterol is subject to more errors and variations than many other lab procedures because cholesterol levels are affected by so many variables such as; stress (both emotional and physical), kidney disease, sleeping problems, infections, gallstones, pancreatic irregularities, diabetes, excessive alcohol, low blood proteins, pregnancy and the use of certain drugs. According to Dr. Pinckney in "The Cholesterol Controversy", fear, anxiety or apprehension at taking such a lab test has been shown to produce a cholesterol level in error by as much as 50 milligrams.

Let's take a look at the animal studies which supposedly "proved" that dietary cholesterol causes heart disease. These studies done in the 1970's used pure isolated cholesterol which had been in bottles on lab shelves for weeks, months or longer. During this long storage period the cholesterol went rancid—that is, oxidized. The researchers were really studying the effects of free radical producing cholesterol—not fresh cholesterol as found in fresh, whole foods. Ten or fifteen years later when these experiments were repeated using fresh, non-oxidized cholesterol the results were much different! Now we have numerous studies which conclusively show that fresh cholesterol does NOT produce the damage to blood vessels that cause atherosclerosis to occur. So why aren't these newer and better studies well publicized? The answer may be a simple matter of economics. Cholesterol testing and management has become a multi-billion dollar profit center for the establishment.

If cholesterol isn't the main cause of heart disease, what is?

If cholesterol isn't the main cause of heart disease, what is?—Atherogenesis, caused by free radical damage in our arteries. The four main culprits are FAT, chlorine in drinking water, smoking and iron overload. There are a great number of other contributors, (see Chapter 1) and the aggregate of all those culprits assure, that most Americans will suffer free radical damage and atherogenesis.

Another interesting fact was revealed by post-mortem studies performed on apparently healthy US soldiers killed in battle during the Korean War. Over 75 percent of these young men, ages 18 to 25, showed "gross evidence of coronary arteriosclerosis", according to the Journal of the American Medical Association. Similar studies during the Vietnam War showed even worse disease. In both cases autopsies performed on enemy soldiers showed no coronary disease. However, there is some very good news that was revealed during and after the war. US prisoners of war that were held captive for three to five years showed a total absence of atherosclerosis. In other words, coronary heart disease is reversible!

While deaths from heart attacks have been decreasing in recent years, cardiovascular disease has not. We seem to be making some progress because of a fairly active public campaign to limit fat consumption, and an even more effective effort against smoking. But, perhaps the main reason heart attack deaths are going down is the massive number of surgical procedures being done. Over 800,000 coronary artery surgeries are performed each year. About half of them are coronary angioplasty and the other half coronary by-pass surgery. Even though these surgeries don't correct the underlying cause they do give many people a chance to change their ways. Within six months stenosis recurs at the site of angioplasty in about 50% of patients. In the other half it takes a year or more. The average cost of angioplasty is $25,000 per artery. The cost of by-pass surgery averages about $125,000.

LEADING CAUSES OF DEATH IN THE U.S.

Rank	Cause of Death	# of Deaths Per Yr.	% of Deaths
1.	Cardio Vascular Disease	940,000	43.2
	Heart Attack	715,000	33.0
	Stroke	150,000	6.9
	Hypertension	30,000	1.4
	Atherosclerosis	24,000	1.1
	Cerebral Hemorrhage	21,000	1.0
2.	Cancer	553,000	25.5
	Lung	132,000	10.4
	Colon	65,000	3.0
	Breast	48,000	2.2
	Prostate	29,000	1.3
	All Other	279,000	12.9
3.	Infectious Diseases	105,000	4.9
	Pneumonia	72,000	3.3
	Aids	16,000	.7
	Influenza	2,000	.1
4.	Accidents	97,000	4.5
	Auto	49,000	2.3
5.	Lung Disease (Not Cancer)	83,000	3.8
6.	Diabetes	40,000	1.9
7.	Suicide	30,500	1.4
8.	Liver Disease	27,000	1.2
9.	Kidney Disease	23,000	1.0
10.	Murder	22,500	1.0

WORDS TO KNOW

Myocardial Infarction

Coronary Thrombosis

Angina Pectoris

Angioplasty

Aneurysms

SUMMARY

1. Heart disease started early in the 1900's. It is a modern day disease.
2. A heart attack is the end result of atherosclerosis, which is the result of free radical damage.
3. Cholesterol has been erroneously named the major cause of heart disease.
4. The good news is that the general disease process that causes cardiovascular disease can be slowed down, stopped and even reversed.
5. Coronary artery surgeries don't cure heart disease, but they do give people time to change their ways.

7

TOO MUCH TOXICITY

In America nearly all of us Love Cars ! ! ! In most families, owning a new car is a very high priority. Among many, having a sexy car is the highest priority.

2 CORINTHIANS 10:2

I beg you that when I come I may not have to be as bold as I expect to be toward some people who think that we live by the standards of this world.

Think for a moment. What kind of car would you really love to drive, a Corvette convertible perhaps, how about a BMW luxury sedan, or maybe that full-time 4 wheel drive Toyota Land Cruiser? There is some car that nearly everyone would dearly love to have.

The next question, of course, is how much are we willing to give up to drive that car? $250 per month? $400 per month? $600 per month? Most people don't have unlimited financial resources so they must prioritize. They must sacrifice something in order to have something else.

Americans buy more new cars than any other nation. There are about two hundred and seventy million people in the U.S. The average family size is about 3, therefore, there are about 90 million families. New car sales in the U.S. are about 10 million per year. Used car sales are nearly double that. The average length of a new car loan is almost 5 years. That means that the average American family is paying for a car all the time. Cars are a very high priority for us it seems.

Let me share some other statistics with you:

- 46 Million Americans have heart disease
- 34% of all Americans will get Cancer

- 21 Million Americans have Diabetes
- 14 Million Americans have severe Arthritis

Let me ask you the same question I asked you in the paragraph above in a little different way. Would you be willing to have Cancer in order to drive that Bemer? Would you take diabetes so you could own a new Chevy? Since there is only so much money to go around, would you give up good health in order to buy that new car? The fact is, most Americans choose to spend their money on 'things' rather than maintaining a high level of health. They would rather buy a new suit than properly feed their "earth suit".

The great majority of Americans are walking, toxic, waste dumps.

Of course, this doesn't come about by a well-thought-out conscious decision to accept a major disease in exchange for the privilege and honor of driving a new car. It is a much more subtle and socially acceptable way of prioritizing our limited resources. We have been taught all of our lives that our modern, scientific, affluent, sedentary lifestyle is not only acceptable but preferable to any other. At the same time, unfortunately, we have not been taught how to properly care for our body. The same philosophy that makes material things a necessity rather than a luxury, has dictated that our health be subordinate to the profits of agri-business, industry, the medical establishment, drug companies, etc. Our educational system is in total concert with this prevailing philosophy, teaching scientifically based absurdities like deadly poison is good for you. In fact, the average American has no idea of his physiology, of how his body works, the pathology of disease, or how to maintain vibrant health.

Controversies abound; Is sugar good for me? Are artificial sweeteners good for me? Is fluoride good for me? Is white flour good for me? Are the drugs I take good for me? Is the water I drink good for me? Are vitamins good for me?

We breathe the air of our polluted atmosphere. We drink the water provided by our local government agency. We eat the food grown by agri-business and processed by huge food companies. For all of the above reasons and many others, the sad fact is, that the great majority of Americans are walking, toxic waste dumps. And poisoning along with malnutrition, are the two major underlying reasons for nearly all degenerative disease.

How Did We Get So Toxic? There are two general areas of concern, environmental toxins and autointoxication (exotoxins and endotoxins).

OUR POLLUTED PLANET

Let's first consider hazardous wastes. According to the 1989 Toxic Release Inventory National Report, U.S. EPA, Office of Toxic Substances:

- 551,000,000 pounds of industrial chemicals were dumped into public sewage systems.
- 1,181,000,000 pounds of chemicals were released into the ground.
- 189,000,000 pounds of chemicals were discharged into surface waters.
- 2,427,000,000 pounds of chemicals were pumped into the atmosphere.
- EPA estimates a grand total of 5,706,000,000 pounds of chemical pollutants were released into the environment.

That's just in one year in the U.S. alone!

How about hazardous waste sites like Love Canal in Niagra Falls, New York? Love Canal has become a national symbol of our hazardous waste problem, as the first mismanaged waste site to be widely recognized. Unfortunately, Love Canal was the first of many! By the 1990's the EPA had identified over 1,000 such sites. Moreover, it is estimated by the EPA, the Office of Technology Assessment, and the Government Accounting Office that many thousands more, uncontrolled hazardous waste sites remain to be found.

And that's just the waste that is recognized as hazardous! America is generating more than six billion tons of "nonhazardous" waste every year.

Besides all of the waste and pollution, products that are obviously toxic, let's enumerate some of the "beneficial chemicals."

Common toxins cause reduced mental functioning, decreased IQ and mental acuity, inability to concentrate and a loss of feeling.

- Chemical Fertilizers
- Pesticides } Farmers have over 50,000
- Insecticides } formulations and 700
- Fungicides } chemical ingredients
- Herbicides } to
- Rodentcides } choose from
- Chlorine in water
- Fluoride
- Food Dyes
- Preservatives
- Artificial Flavors
- Artificial Sweeteners
- Cleaning Chemicals
- Over-the-Counter Medications
- Prescription Drugs

Since the discovery of the insecticidal properties of DDT in 1942, vast quantities of chlorinated hydrocarbons have been sprayed over the surface of the earth in an effort to destroy insects. These efforts initially met with good success, however, we now know of their harmful, even tragic, side effects.

Chlorohydrocarbons are highly stable compounds and can remain in the environment for decades. They are also fat soluble and accumulate in the tissues of most animals, especially animals at the top of the food chain, including man.

Estimates indicate that about one billion pounds of DDT were spread throughout the world ecosystem, with many pronounced detrimental effects. One effect is that it inhibits the enzyme carbonic anhydrase that controls the calcium supply for egg shell formation in most birds. In the decades following the 1940's the population of eagles, falcons and hawks dropped dramatically. There is no doubt that DDT was responsible.

Although DDT has been outlawed in the U.S. and many other nations, it is still used in relatively minor amounts. Unfortunately, there are literally hundreds of new poisons being sprayed with yet unknown side effects.

The entire medical field is functionally illiterate on the subject of low-level toxicology.

In his book, *Diet for a Poisoned Planet*, David Steinman says, "Cancer, Alzheimer's Disease, Parkinson's Disease and Heart Disease are late consequences of exposure. Researchers on the cutting edge of chemical toxicology have established that among the first consequences of exposure to common toxic chemicals is neurotoxicity: **reduced mental functioning, decreased IQ and mental acuity, inability to concentrate, and loss of feeling.** Cancer, which has gotten much of the attention, is one of the last consequences to appear. Other insidious conditions include **diabetes, Epstein-Barr Syndrome, Chronic Fatigue Syndrome, weakened immunity and anxiety."**

Unfortunately, the medical community is of little help in these areas. They have little training in chemical toxicology. The expert committee of the National Academy of Sciences in its landmark 1988 publication *Role of the Primary Care Physician in Occupational Environmental Medicine*, concluded that the entire medical field is functionally illiterate on the subject of the low-level toxicology of industrial pollution, pesticides and food additives.

There has been so much literature published on pollution, that the American public seems to have become immune to it. Or, maybe it is just the general consensus of American thought. Like the time a nutritional activist was giving a talk on this very subject, he said to the audience, "It seems like the average

American is both ignorant of, and apathetic about, the environmental pollution problem." He then turned to a man on the front row and asked what he thought. The man replied, "I don't know and I don't care."

INTERNAL POLLUTION

"In treating over 300,000 patients, it is the bowel that invariably has to be cared for first, before any effective healing can take place."

Unfortunately, environmental pollution and toxicity is just part of the problem. A malfunctioning digestive system caused by our prevailing lifestyle and eating habits is also part of our toxic problem.

Many health experts agree that getting rid of waste products and toxins, particularly from our digestive tract, is prerequisite to good health.

Dr. Norman W. Walker in *Colon Health*, "The fact of the matter is that constipation is the number one affliction underlying nearly every ailment; it can be imputed to be the initial, primary cause of nearly every disturbance of the human system."

Dr. Bernard Jensen in *Tissue Cleansing Through Bowel Management*, "In the 50 years I've spent helping people to overcome illness, disability and disease, it has become crystal clear that poor bowel management lies at the root of most people's health problems. In treating over 300,000 patients, it is the bowel that invariably has to be cared for first, before any effective healing can take place."

V.E. Irons in *The Destruction of Your Own Natural Protective Mechanism*, "It is probably too late to save our Nation but we can save thousands of individuals who can see and believe in our theory that the cause of most conditions of ill health is autointoxication and that 95% of their troubles start in the colon.

Dr. John Harvey Kellog, Robert Gray, Dr. Paavo Airola, and many other health experts say essentially the same thing; most diseases start in the colon. Even if all these men were only half right, the colon would still be a very important organ to maintain for a healthy body.

The colon or bowel or large intestine is about 5 to 6 feet long and connects the small intestine with the anus. It should be between 2 and $2^1/_2$ inches in diameter and weigh about $1^1/_2$ pounds. During autopsies, when an examiner removes and inspects the different organs of the body to find the reasons for the death of the individual, it is not unusual to find colons 5, 6 or 7 inches in diameter and weighing 12, 15 or even 20 pounds. In extreme cases colons have been found to be 12 inches in diameter and weigh 50 pounds. Can you imagine having 50 pounds of aging, rotten, putrid fecal material in your body? The major function of the colon, of course, is the elimination of waste products from the body. There are several other functions: a) a properly functioning colon will reabsorb about 70% of the water passing through it, b) friendly bacteria in the colon manufacture enzymes and vitamins such as B12. (Maybe you've heard that you must get B12 from eating meat. From 85% to 100% of B12 in meat is killed during cooking), c) the lymph system "back flushes" into the colon. A clogged colon means an overloaded lymph system.

Can you imagine having many pounds of aging, rotten, putrid, fecal material in your body

The colon is a mucous membrane organ. When everything is working properly the colon has the right amount of mucous in the correct consistency. However, eating the average American diet, this is seldom the case. Certain foods and pollutants cause the production of large amounts of sticky mucous (the FDA has allowed over 10,000 different chemicals to be added to our food). This sticky mucous is designed to protect the body from these ingested toxins. This process would work fine if it happened once a month or even once a week, but we usually eat chemicals and mucoid producing foods with every meal and snack. So, rather than normal mucous we get too much sticky mucous, which slows things down, which causes a tendency towards constipation. To complicate things, we don't eat enough fiber. Fiber retains moisture and provides bulk for the colon to push against. The lack of fiber, therefore, also causes a tendency toward constipation.

Of course, we Americans eat way too much salt, which dries out tissue, particularly smooth muscle. Smooth muscle is the kind that makes up those muscular tubes we call arteries, and the intestine, and provides the peristaltic action that moves the fecal material through the colon. Too much salt reduces this peristaltic action, causing a tendency toward constipation.

If we ate the way the Bible tells us to eat we would be getting about 15% protein, 15% fat and 70% complex carbohydrates. Unfortunately, the American diet contains 30% to 40% protein, 40% to 50% fat, way too much simple carbohydrates, and of course, not nearly enough complex carbohydrates. Grains, beans, fruits and vegetables are complex carbohydrates and are whole live foods. They contain lots of nutrients in the proper ratios (vitamins, minerals, enzymes, fatty acids, amino acids, etc.), lots of dietary fiber, lots of available energy, and very few calories. This is so important to the colon, and therefore the entire body, because the kind of bacteria that break down carbohydrates—the Good Guys—are different than the bacteria that break down fats and proteins—the Bad Guys. The best known Good Guy is lactobacillus acidophilus and the best known Bad Guy is bacillus coli. The function of the Good Guys is to decompose carbohydrates, and the by-products of that function are vitamins and enzymes. The function of the Bad Guys is to break down fat and protein and the by-products of that function are toxins and poisons.

The healthy intestinal wall is lined with hundreds of different varieties of microorganisms that number in the billions. Some are good, friendly bacteria while others are unhealthful. When the "good" bacteria outnumber the "bad" by 3 to 1, or 4 to 1, there is likely to be good intestinal health and a properly functioning lower G.I. tract. This rich protective coating of microorganisms work together with the cells making up the lining of the intestinal tract to protect our body from unhealthy bacteria, yeast, wastes, toxins and chemicals; while at the same time allowing life-giving water and nutrients to be absorbed into circulation, taken to the liver, and feed every cell in our body.

Besides the friendly bacteria, our body provides a number of functions to do battle against the unhealthful bacteria. Lactoferrin, for example, is a protein that traps iron so it can't be used by bad bacteria. Without iron the bad bacteria will weaken and die. Globulin proteins prevent bad bacteria from adhering to the intestine wall, thus being eliminated with the feces. Lactoperoxidase is an enzyme that attacks and damages bad bacteria.

In spite of all the body tries to do, so many times the unhealthful bacteria overpower the good and proliferate. When this happens toxins are manufactured, yeast and parasites thrive, the semi-permeability of the intestinal wall is changed into a sieve and toxins, waste and other filth pour into the liver.

Too often, toxins, waste and other filth pour into the liver.

There are a number of factors that in combination can lead to excessive and inappropriate permeability of the colonic membrane.

1) Chronic nutritional insufficiency
2) Irritation of the gut lining
3) Imbalance or overgrowth of intestinal flora
4) Circulating bacterial produced toxins
5) Nonsteroidal anti-inflammatory drugs such as ibuprofen and aspirin (NSAIDS)

Ironically, many people who have an inflammatory disease are prescribed NSAIDS for the inflammation and pain relief, which may exaggerate the problems of both gut permeability and the inflammatory disease itself.

According to Dr. John Harvey Kellog, this country's foremost pioneer of colon health, the bacteria in a healthy colon ideally should be 85% lactobacteria and no more than 15% coliform bacteria. Unfortunately, in our society those numbers are reversed. No wonder the misery caused by autointoxication is so great and the problems with flatulence are so frequent.

Autointoxication occurs when the toxins and poisons produced by the bad bacteria attack the semi-permeable membrane of the colon causing it to malfunction in its discriminating capacity. That is, to allow the bad things (toxins and poisons) to be absorbed along with the water and vitamins and enzymes. Because of our diet then, we have a tendency toward constipation and the proliferation of bad bacteria which causes autointoxication not to mention an environment which encourages parasites.

Because of our diet, we have a tendency toward constipation and the proliferation of bad bacteria which causes autointoxication.

What makes autointoxication so bad is where these toxins and poisons are taken when they are absorbed into our system. You see, there are veins throughout the digestive tract that pick up everything that is absorbed from the colon and small intestine. These veins flow into larger and larger tributaries until they all come into one large vein known as the portal vein. The portal vein's destination is the liver. The liver is supposed to be the recipient of all that pure water, vitamins, minerals and enzymes that were absorbed from our food. But along with the water and nutrients, the liver receives toxins and poisons produced by the coliform bacteria as well as large quantities of putrid filth and fecal material that the colon can't get rid of in the normal way.

When you realize that the liver performs more functions than all of the other organs combined and that regeneration of every part of the body starts in the liver, then you can begin to understand why so many health experts agree that so much illness and disease starts in the colon.

On top of all that, when the colon isn't working properly the lymph system can't perform properly causing problems in the immune system. A weak immune system allows an increase in the probability of infections, allergies, cancer and other ailments.

So, what should be done? First, of course, we should change our dietary habits to treat the colon kindly. Second, consider a colon cleansing program to overcome the effects of the years of abusive eating and other colon neglect. Please don't use laxatives on a regular basis. What happens when a laxative is taken? The result is usually the ejection of debris from the colon. But why did this take place? Simply because the colon became so irritated in expelling the offending laxative that some other loose material went out with it. Laxatives and cathartics are not only habit-forming but decidedly destructive to the intestines.

THE PROCESS OF DETOXIFICATION

Because of pollution, our prevailing lifestyle and eating habits, most of us need detoxifying from time to time, while some need detoxifying before health can return.

The following is the average unhealthy scenario of toxicity:

Step 1: Toxins enter the body, while other toxins and poisons are formed internally, leak through the malfunctioning intestine and are taken to the liver.

Step 2: Toxins are not completely detoxified in an unhealthy liver.

Step 3: Toxins leave the liver and are stored in tissues like fat, the brain and nervous system.

Step 4: Stored toxins recirculate in the blood, contributing to long term, poor health.

The following is how detoxification is designed to work:

Step 1: Toxins enter the body. In the healthy digestive system few poisons are formed and most toxins are excreted, with only small amounts reaching the liver.

Step 2: The healthy liver transforms toxins into intermediate substances.

Step 3: Harmful free radicals are formed as a result of Step 2, but are rendered harmless by our body's antioxidant defenses.

Step 4: The healthy liver changes the intermediate substances into harmless water soluble substances that are released through the kidneys as urine.

Your body knows when it can safely detox and when it should store toxins instead.

The most difficult toxins for the body to eliminate are the non-polar, lipid-soluble type. These molecules are generally stored in our adipose (fat) tissue, many times for a considerable length of time before the body can convert and eliminate them. DDT for example can remain in an unhealthy body for years.

The liver converts toxic substances into more polar, water-soluble compounds using two broad steps. In phase one, a super family of enzymes known as the Cytochrome P450 system, reduce, oxidize or hydrolyze the toxins. The intermediate metabolites produced in the first step are then attacked by other liver enzymes to form much less harmful chemicals like sulfates, glutathione adducts, and other conjugates that are eliminated in the urine or feces.

It is critically important that both steps work together because the intermediate metabolites produced in the first step many times are actually more harmful than the original toxins. In addition, the first step produces many free radicals such as superoxide anion radical, hydroxyl radical and others. So, if the second set of liver enzymes are inadequate or the antioxidant defenses are lacking, detoxification can make people feel worse, while leading to free radical pathology and disease. Your body knows when it can safely detox and when it should store toxins instead.

The most popular methods (but potentially harmful) used to detoxify the colon, liver, etc. are forcing laxatives or herbs and fasting. The detoxifying process is not only highly energy intensive but is also dependent on sufficient antioxidant nutrients as well as adequate levels of other supporting nutrients. Therefore, a broad based nutritional approach is advantageous for a number of reasons; gives optimum liver enzyme support, prevents muscle tissue catabolism, stabilizes blood sugar levels and protects against free radical damage.

There are a great number of colon cleansing programs, liver cleansing products, and tissue cleaning and detoxifying programs on the market. Most of them FORCE the body to begin cleansing with severely inadequate nutritional support. Depending on the condition of the participant, the results can be dangerous. But, that may not be the worst part. The worst part may be embracing the same philosophy to get us out of trouble that got us in trouble in the first place. We need to change from the prevailing "figure-it-out-and-force-the-body-back-to-health" philosophy to a philosophy of allowing our bodies to rebuild better health by following proper principles, by following God's recommendations on eating and lifestyle.

While fasting is wonderful in several ways, a nutrient supported cleansing fast may be the most effective, least expensive and least hazardous method to detoxify and thereby quickly gain a higher level of health.

WORDS TO KNOW

Autointoxication	Portal Vein
Lactobacteria	Detoxify

SUMMARY

1. Americans have been taught to spend most of their limited financial resources on "things" and not on good health.
2. Even the most straight forward and obvious health issues are clouded tremendously by controversy.
3. Most Americans are toxic.
4. Toxicity comes from our polluted environment—exotoxins and autointoxication—endotoxins.
5. Toxins are stored in fat, brain and nerve tissue.
6. Neurotoxicity is affecting most Americans with reduced mental functioning, decreased I.Q., inability to concentrate, chronic fatigue, Epstein-Barr, etc.
7. Many toxic problems start in the colon because of incomplete digestion and elimination.
8. Toxins and poisons are detoxified in the liver.
9. Forced detoxification can be dangerous.
10. Detoxification uses lots of energy and nutrients.
11. A nutrient supported cleansing fast may be the safest way to quickly promote better health through elimination of toxins.

YOUTHFULNESS

Youth is not only a time of life, it is a state of mind. Youth means the predominance of courage over timidity, of adventure over ease. It means the lure of wonder, the appetite for what's next, and a joy for living. Toxicity may be the main enemy of youth. So, let's all improve our attitudes, eat real foods and die young at any age!

8

SMOKING

I CORINTHIANS 6:12

Everything is permissible for me—but not everything is beneficial. Everything is permissible for me—I will not be mastered by anything.

Chemical carcinogens have been widely publicized as health hazards for smokers. So we will just touch on this lightly. Nicotine, of course, is a poisonous drug, but smoking also introduces two other deadly poisons into your body-arsenic and carbon monoxide. Smoking constricts the capillaries of the air sacs, impairing the flow of blood, it also causes them to lose their elasticity. Tobacco neutralizes vitamin C and of course causes emphysema and cancer. But now research focuses on radioactivity: The New-found danger in cigarettes!

We live on a planet with low levels of natural radioactivity from such sources as cosmic rays, but with each cigarette, a smoker inhales almost as much polonium-210 as he would get from natural sources in 24 hours. Thus the average smoker exposes himself each day to about 30 times more of this long-lived radioactive element than do most non-smokers.

In the evening, after a hard day of work, a smoker lights up. For years he has done this, enjoying the puff and the smoke and the glow, though dimly aware of publicity about chemical hazards. But if his eyes could detect what scientific instruments can, he would see radioactivity coming from his cigarette and from his body — from his lungs, liver, kidneys, pancreas, sex glands and even from the bones of his skeleton.

Can this radioactivity in cigarettes cause cancer? When a smoker lights up, he inhales more than 4,000 chemicals with his first puff. Some, such as the polycyclic aromatic hydrocarbon benzo(a)pyrene, are powerful carcinogens. When Dr. Little and his Harvard colleagues exposed animals sequentially to alpha radiation from polonium-210 and to benzo(a)pyrene, they found that the two substances together acted synergistically and caused malignant lung tumors at "about twice the rate expected from the simple additive effect" of polonium-210 and benzo(a)pyrene.

180,000 Americans are estimated to die each year from smoking-related cancers.

Radioactive elements in cigarette smoke can also accumulate in areas important to a body's immune defenses. There is evidence indicating that smoking can undermine the body's ability to fight off poisons, cancer and other diseases.

Cigarettes contain so much radioactivity, according to Dr. Thomas H. Winters, director of an occupational health center in North Quincy, Mass., and Dr. Joseph R. DiFranza of the University of Massachusetts Medical Center, that a pack-and-a-half-per-day smoker gets a yearly dose of radiation in parts of his lungs equal to what his skin would be exposed to in about 300 chest X rays. Scientists are only beginning to discover how much harm the radioactive isotopes in cigarettes do. Estimates vary dramatically as to the number of cases of lung cancer in smokers that are caused by radiation in cigarettes. Dr. DiFranza, however, believes that "radiation alone could account for about half of all lung cancers in smokers." 180,000 Americans are estimated to die each year from smoking-related cancers—most from lung cancer.

Radioactive Footprints. How did radioactive elements get into cigarettes? T.C. Tso, a former researcher for the U.S. Department of Agriculture, tracked these radioactive footprints to the fields where tobacco is grown. For many decades, farmers have fertilized tobacco crops with phosphates rich in uranium. By decay, this uranium generates radium-226, which in turn spawns radon-222, and eventually lead-210 and polonium-210. Tobacco plants readily absorb radioactive elements from the fertilizer and from naturally occurring radiation in the soil, air and water. Breezes and farm equipment whip these dangerous elements into the air, where they are absorbed by the sticky resin tips of hairs that grow on each tobacco leaf.

When a smoker lights up, the heat of the cigarette's glowing tip fires the hair tips of the tobacco into insoluble particles, which, incorporating the radioactive isotopes, are then inhaled deep into the smoker's lungs. Inside the lungs the airways branch out into smaller and smaller passageways. It is especially at each branching, many scientists claim, that the particles in the inhaled smoke tend to accumulate, much as floating river debris piles up on sand bars.

As a smoker consumes cigarette after cigarette, these particles may be deposited at the same points in the lungs. According to Edward A. Martell, a specialist in radiochemistry at the National Center for Atmospheric Research, these points become "hot spots" of radioactivity. Martell believes it is no coincidence that most lung cancers begin at these branch points where radioactive debris gathers.

A healthy body's defenses are usually able to clear away the smoke, ash and poison-gas pollution from a single cigarette within hours. But the accumulated smoke particles are much harder to remove from the moist protective coating of lung tissues, the bronchial epithelium, and remain in the lungs usually for three to six months, in some instances for many years—emitting radiation.

Eventually the body's immune-system cells clean these particles from the lungs, but in the process the radioisotopes are carried into the bloodstream and to other parts of the body—the liver, pancreas, kidneys, lymph nodes, thyroid and bone marrow. Here, too, the radioactive particles accumulate year after year, emitting radiation that can damage nearby cells.

Martell notes that the calcified plaques in the blood vessels of smokers suffering atherosclerosis (hardening of the arteries) show high levels of lead-210 and polonium-210, the same radioactive isotopes inhaled with tobacco smoke—and he speculates that the radiation in cigarettes may also be a contributing factor in smokers' developing atherosclerosis, which itself can lead to early coronaries and also to strokes.

Dangerous Interaction. How long does such radioactivity persist in a smoker's body? Radioactive lead-210 has a half-life of 21.4 years. Beverly S. Cohen and Naomi H. Harley of the New York University Medical Center discovered that smokers who quit still had, five years later, almost as much lower-lung radioactivity from lead-210 as did active smokers. And most smokers do not quit permanently. Indeed, each year the average smoker in the United States consumes more than 11,000 cigarettes.

Alpha radiation smashes into atoms, turning them into ions that can readily damage the genetic blueprint of living cells.

The most harmful radiation in cigarettes, however, comes not from lead-210, which emits the relatively weak beta radiation, but from its radioactive 'granddaughter,' polonium-210, which emits highly localized, ionizing alpha radiation, the same sort given off by the plutonium of atom bombs. Alpha radiation smashes into atoms, turning them into ions that can readily damage the genetic blueprint of living cells, killing them or turning them into cancer cells. Scientists have recognized the danger to living things in beta radiation, but alpha radiation can be 20 times as damaging.

Menace in the Home. Recently scientists discovered another deadly mixture in smoking. Soil gives off small amounts of radon, a radioactive gas derived from radium. New weather-sealing technologies to help conserve energy in our homes can also trap and concentrate this dangerous gas indoors. The Environmental Protection Agency estimates that up to 20,000 Americans each year may be dying from lung cancer caused by inhaling radon in homes and work places.

But when indoor air already polluted with invisible, odorless radon gas is also polluted with cigarette smoke, something even more frightening happens. In clean air the radon's short-lived daughters tend to attach themselves to walls, rugs and draperies. But with tobacco smoke in the air, the radon daughters condense onto smoke particles and remain aloft to be inhaled by smokers and those who breathe secondhand smoke. As a result, the combination of indoor radon pollution and indoor cigarette-smoke pollution may create yet another synergy deadlier than each of the pollutants separately.

Even without radon, those who breathe smoke-clouded air will be dosed with radioactivity from tobacco. At least 50 percent of the radioactive isotopes in cigarette smoke wind up in the air, and a smaller percentage of this and other elements in the smoke are inhaled by those around the smoker. Dr. Takeshi Hirayama of the Institute of Preventive Oncology in Tokyo studied records of more than 91,000 women and found that non-smoking wives of heavy smokers had more than double the risk of dying from lung cancer than did the non-smoking wives of non-smokers.

With all that scientists have learned about radioactivity in cigarettes, they say that the best way to protect yourself is not to let tobacco smoke into your lungs at all.

Everyone now knows that smoking is very dangerous to our health. Even the tobacco companies have, at long last, been forced to admit this and accept part of the financial responsibility as a result of recent litigation and out-of-court settlements.

If you still smoke—**STOP!**

If you can't stop—**CONTINUE TO TRY TO STOP!**

Don't light up... for just one more hour... And then another... And another...

If you are a Christian, ask yourself this question, "How does smoking bring glory to God?"

WORDS TO KNOW

Radioactive

Polonium-210

Isotopes

Alpha Radiation

Radon

SUMMARY

1. Tobacco smoke contains more than 4,000 chemicals, many being cancer causing like benzo(a)pyrene. Other poisons include arsenic, carbon monoxide and nicotine.
2. The other half of the smoking problem is the large concentration of cancer causing radioactive elements like polonium-210.
3. When poisonous chemical carcinogens team up with radioactive isotopes the cancer causing effects are greatly enhanced.

9

FLUORIDE

ANOTHER DECISION YOU WILL HAVE TO MAKE

For those of us who have decided to take responsibility for our own health, whether or not to avoid fluoride is another decision we will have to make. Notice the decision is to "avoid" fluoride NOT whether to use it! That's because if you don't make a conscious effort to avoid fluoride, the decision has already been made for you. Let's look at some of the facts about fluoride and see if you agree with this decision that has been made for you and your children. Remember, to the apathetic goes the fluoride.

PROVERBS 14:7

Stay away from a foolish man, for you won't find knowledge on his lips.

In the United States the population as a whole is kept ignorant of any adverse effect that might occur from exposure to fluorides. In fact, fluorides are touted as beneficial, "good for our teeth". However, fluorides are high on the SUPERFUND PRIORITIES LIST of 275 toxic chemical substances which pose the most significant risk to human health. By Public Law 99-499, the Agency for Toxic Substances and Disease Registry is required to publish a toxicological profile for fluorides and update the document every three years. The April 1993 Toxicological Profile for Fluorides, Hydrogen Fluoride and Fluorine (F) establishes that exposure to fluorides do, in fact, cause harm to the population in general and particularly to vulnerable subsets of the population.

WHAT IS A FLUORIDE?

ALL FLUORIDES ARE POISON

By definition, fluorides are the product of the element fluorine combined with another element or elements. Fluorine is the most corrosive, reactive, oxidizing and electronegative of all the elements. That means that fluorine radically changes everything it touches. For example, when you expose water to a stream of fluorine, the water will burn! Because it is so corrosive, fluorine is never found in its pure state in nature — it is always combined with something.

In addition, fluorine is the most toxic member of the halogen family and second only to arsenic on the scale of toxicity. Fluorine is also well known for its ability to work with other poisons and medicines and drugs to make them much stronger and much worse. For example, Sarin, a nerve gas, one of the most potent fluorine based compounds is so toxic it requires just .001 parts per billion to kill a man.

Of course, some fluorides are much more toxic than others. In general, the more soluble the fluoride, the more toxic it is. For example, calcium and magnesium fluorides found in naturally fluoridated water are less soluble and reactive than fluoride compounds used for artificial drinking water fluoridation. Compounds like oxygen difluoride, chlorine trifluoride and related structures are strong oxidizers and are highly destructive to living organisms both via chemical reaction with tissue and by poisoning of numerous body enzymes. In other words, fluorides are both poison and free radicals.

If a person would get a lot of fluoride all at once the acute toxic poisoning would happen immediately and the effects would be known. However, with prolonged low-level exposure, the cause and effect is usually not apparent and is almost always attributed to other factors. The average person is much more likely to suffer from the effects of long term, low-level fluoride intoxication. Consequently, the symptoms are confused with other common diseases for which the recommended medicine is often a fluorine-based medication like Prozac or fluacizine.

There are a number of recent scientific studies that show fluorides to be aggressive neurotoxins. On page 125 of the government toxicity profile referred to earlier it says, "Neurotoxicity... Because fluoride interacts with calcium ions needed for effective neurotransmission, fluoride can effect the nervous system." Other studies indicate the brain is a target organ of fluoride, in particular, the hippocampus (learning center) seems to be greatly effected. The hippocampus is our central processor which integrates input from our surroundings, from our memory and from our motivation to produce behavior and to remember things. So, the bottom line is that fluoride seems to contribute to motor-sensory dysfunction, IQ deficits, learning disabilities and hyperactivity. To make things worse, most of the psychoactive (mental function changing) drugs like hypnotics, stimulants, antidepressants, anesthetics, and sleeping aids are fluoride based.

Many scientists are concerned about fluoride's effect on our glands, particularly the thyroid gland.

Many chemists and scientists are concerned about fluoride's effect on our glands, particularly the thyroid gland. There is a law of chemistry called halogen displacement. This law says that all five halogens can displace an element with a higher atomic weight. The atomic weight of fluorine is 19 while that of iodine is 127. Iodine is essential for thyroid function. A poorly functioning thyroid effects our metabolism and can cause chronic fatigue and/or hyperactivity. And, of course, proper weight management is an important function of the thyroid.

The proponents of fluoride quote a lot of scientific studies also. In reading these studies it quickly becomes apparent that they don't really compare to the real world we live in. Animal studies use pedigreed, virus-free, disease resistant animals, fed special diets and distilled water and given high-grade sodium fluoride in controlled doses.

In real life most people don't eat or drink properly nor are we perfectly healthy. We are exposed to a variety of fluorides in combination with other poisons and chemicals. For example, most municipal water systems that fluoridate their water use fluorosilicates, which is a toxic waste product from pollution scrubbing operations of phosphate fertilizer manufacturing facilities. Unlike the pharmaceutical grade sodium fluoride used for clinical research, the industrial waste fluorides are contaminated with mercury, cadmium, lead, arsenic, uranium, polonium, radium and radon among others. In Florida, which is a major source for fluorisilicates used for water fluoridation, the phosphate rock contains about 3 1/2% total fluorine and about 300 parts per million of uranium oxide. Significant alpha radiation (the kind that causes cancer in people) is emitted by this radioactive material, but manufacturers are not required to monitor radio nuclide levels.

An example of synergistic toxicity of fluorides is when Dupont's fungicide Benlate DF was accidentally contaminated with a fluoride-based fungicide, Flusilazole. (Flusilazole can't be used in the United States but is sold overseas). Benlate alone is so powerful it takes just one thimble full to treat one acre of land. The combination, however, created a super mutagen which was found toxic at parts per trillion. In fact, it required the development of special equipment because toxic levels were so minute. The Haz-Mat teams removing the contaminated dirt from the farms became seriously ill even though they were wearing protective gear and were properly decontaminated. Since the average person gets fluoride from a variety of sources the toxic combinations that can occur in our bodies is simply unknown.

SOURCES OF FLUORIDE

The studies that proclaim fluoride to be not only safe but beneficial, only consider the amount a person would get by drinking fluoridated water. However, there are a number of other sources of fluoride for the average person.

1. Fluoridated Water—about 2 mg per day
2. Normal food sources—between 2 and 3 mg per day

3. Tooth brushing—between 2 and 3 mg per day
4. Residual fluorides from pesticides, fungicides and herbicides. For example, some fruit juices contain over 6 mg of fluorides per liter
5. Fluoridated mouth rinses, gels and dental floss
6. Processed foods and beverages made with fluoridated water
7. Cooking with fluoridated water. Heat also affects how fluorides react with other chemicals like food preservatives and chlorine
8. Fluoride based drugs and medicines
9. Fluoride treatments in dentists' offices and schools
10. Fluoride supplements
11. Fluoride added to bottled water

How much is enough? How much is too much? Many proponents of fluoride mistakenly say that fluoride is a nutrient or essential element. This is simply not true. According to a report in 1989 by the National Academy of Sciences, fluorides are not nutrients nor are they essential for human development.

It would be quite interesting to describe how fluoride effects your DNA, your enzymes, your functions, your organs and glands in great scientific detail, but that is beyond the scope of this book. Just a quick sentence or two will give you an idea. Molecules in our body are held together by chemical bonds. There are a number of kinds of chemical bonds like, anionic bonds, covalent bonds, hydrogen bonds and many others. In our bodies our nucleic acids and enzymes use a lot of hydrogen bonds to stay together and function properly. Fluorides break these hydrogen bonds in our RNA, DNA and enzymes causing our cells to malfunction and sometimes to mutate.

FOR THOSE WHO WOULD LIKE TO LEARN MORE, CONSIDER THE FOLLOWING WORKS:

Fluoride the Aging Factor, by John Yiamouyiannis, Ph.D.

Fluoridation the Great Delemma, by George L. Waldbott, M.D.

How to Save Your Teeth - Toxic - Free Preventive Dentistry, by David Kennedy, D.D.S.

Fluoride: A toxic Tort Perspective - Panacea or Poison, by George C. Glasser

WORDS TO KNOW

Neurotoxicity

Hippocampus

Psychoactive

Radioactive

SUMMARY

1. Fluorine is the most corrosive element in nature, and the second most toxic element in nature.
2. Most fluorides are strong, free radicals to our tissues and extremely poisonous to our bodies' nucleic acids and enzymes.
3. Fluorides are also aggressive neurotoxins.
4. Most people suffer from long term low level fluoride intoxication, therefore, the symptoms are confused with other diseases.
5. Fluorides are most often contaminated with other toxic chemicals like mercury, cadmium, lead, arsenic, uranium, polonium, radium and radon.
6. Today the unsuspecting public gets way too much fluoride from a variety of sources.

10

SOME LIKE IT SWEET

We will be spending most of our time in this chapter talking about two villains, sugar and Aspartame, and one "good guy," stevia.

TITUS 3:3

At one time we too were foolish, dis-obedient, deceived and enslaved by all kinds of passions and pleasures

Sugar is by far the most popular sweetener, so it deserves to be mentioned first. What is sugar anyway, and how do we get it?

The chemical name of refined sugar is Sucrose ($C_{12}H_{22}O_{11}$). Sucrose is a disaccharide. That means it is made up of two Saccharides called fructose and glucose ($C_6H_{12}O_6$). Glucose is the primary source of fuel used by our body to make energy. Another name for Saccharides is carbohydrates. There are many different kinds of Saccharides like monosaccharides, disaccharides and polysaccharides. Monosaccharides and disacharides are simple carbohydrates or sugars while polysacharides are complex carbohydrates. Complex carbohydrates are what our bodies need the most, while simple carbohydrates (sugars) can turn destructive in a hurry.

Since every plant contains carbohydrates, it would be possible to refine sugar from any plant, but some are much better than others for this purpose—cane, beets and corn. The objective of the refining process is to isolate the sugar from everything else in the plant and make it attractive for sale. In other words, refining makes sugar pure and white. Obviously, all nutrients are removed during this process.

The refining process for beets would go something like this. Sugar beets must first be juiced by slicing them and treating them with hot water. Lime is mixed with the extracted juice and then exposed to burning sulphur fumes. It's next washed in a centrifuge with salts of tin and blueing and acid phosphates. Finally it goes to a filter press and after evaporation what is left is bleached.

At this point sugar can only be called food because it contains calories, but it certainly does not contain any nutrients. Refined sugar is bad for us for a multitude of reasons. The number one reason is because we eat so much of it. The average American eats about 165 pounds of sugar every year. That equals out to 68 teaspoons of sugar every day.

As you can see, the following advertisement is promoting sugar as a wonderful low calorie food, just 16 calories per teaspoon. Let's see, 16 calories times 68 teaspoons—that's 1088 calories. So the average American eats over 1000 empty, that is, nutrition-free, calories every day. Anyone watching their weight?

The Sugar Association, based in Washington, D.C. ran the following magazine ad a couple of years ago. I've kept it because I find some of its statements fascinating, like, "... sugar comes naturally from either sugar cane or sugar beets". Read the refining process on sugar beets included in this discussion and decide for yourself if that process is natural.

Is Someone Trying to silence the truth about sugar?

It's quite mysterious, but someone is trying to misinform America about real sugar. By popularizing misconceptions and perpetuating myths. By slanting the truth.

Who could be doing this? The users of cheaper substitute sweeteners, like corn syrup? Misguided health and diet faddists? Artificial sweetener manufacturers? Self-proclaimed "experts" who knock sugar to promote useless foods and diets? We think it's time you knew the real truth about real sugar.

Sugar is a natural food.

Unlike artificial sweeteners that contain man-made chemicals, real sugar comes naturally from either sugar cane or sugar beets. Not from a laboratory. In fact, sugar is an important member of the carbohydrate family which is used by the body to provide energy.

Sugar isn't high in calories.

Actually it contains a lot less calories than most people suspect; only 16 calories per teaspoon.

Sugar is safe.

Artificial sweeteners are required to have warning labels. You'll never find a warning label on sugar. The Food and Drug Administration has placed sugar on its "Generally Recognized as Safe" list. No artificial sweetener is on this list. None.

Sugar tastes best.

Quite simply, sugar is good food...good for your body and good to your taste buds. It remains unmatched in taste. Unmatched in quality. Real sugar has always been the best. It still is.

Real Sugar

It's always been the best. It still is.

How about this statement, "Sugar isn't high in calories." Hmm, "high" is a relative term, but over 1000 calories from sugar each day seems pretty high to me.

Finally, "Quite simply, sugar is good food..." I don't even consider sugar a food, let alone good! But then I am one of those misguided health faddists "perpetuating myths" and "slanting the truth." There is, however, one statement I agree with, I also... "think it is time you knew the real truth about real sugar."

Sugar is a major factor in malnutrition

Another major problem with sugar is that it uses up a lot of nutrients in our body, things like Thiamin (B1), Calcium, Chromium and others. When you eat a food like fruit, you will be getting some sugar, of course, but that apple or banana also contains all the nutrients needed to utilize the sugar properly. When you eat refined sugar, your body must supply those nutrients.

For example, both Thiamin and Chromium are necessary to metabolize sugar. When we use up a lot of the body's Thiamin for processing sugar, that throws the B complex off balance. The B complex vitamins are known as the 'stress' vitamins. Think there might be a connection? Chromium is used in the production of insulin. Insulin is what moves sugar out of the blood. Low chromium often means diabetes.

Sugar is a major factor in malnutrition. There are three reasons for this:

1. Sugar itself is nutrition-free.
2. Sugar demands the body to use up many nutrients.
3. Sugar decreases the desire to eat wholesome foods.

Sugar promotes restless, aggressive and destructive behavior and shows up as learning disorders like Attention Deficit Disorder, (ADD). Eating sugar causes our body to make endorphins. Under normal conditions endorphins are good. They are natural pain killers. In fact, they do the same thing to us as heroin. Both endorphins and heroin are narcotics called opiates. They are central nervous system depressants. Since opiates are depressants, developing tolerance to them shows up as nervous system excitement or tension. This feeling of tension is exactly what a drug addict feels during withdrawal—a craving for the drug.

Of course, our natural opiates are produced by our body in much smaller quantities than a heroin user would give himself. None the less, the feelings and effects are the same, just not in the same magnitude. Add to this the fact that toxins are stored in brain and nerve tissue, and the generally poor eating habits of the average student, and it's pretty clear why Ritalin is now the most prescribed drug, by far, for American children.

Sugar promotes restless, aggressive and destructive behavior and shows up as learning disorders like ADD.

Sugar is not a good food! Some say sugar is not a food at all, however, it will be found in most processed foods you can buy. Only salt appears on more ingredient lists. I would like to develop the history of sugar, how the demand for it promoted mass kidnappings, hundreds of thousands of murders and slavery in the new world, among other things. Sugar certainly contributes greatly to the poor health and reduced mental capacity of untold millions of people, especially our children. Sounds like a satanic scheme to me. However, this is not a history text so we will leave the curious to search it out for themselves.

ASPARTAME

As bad as sugar is, it is probably better to eat it, rather than artificial sweeteners. First, there was cyclamate; banned because it caused cancer. Then came saccharine, which is still with us but carries a warning label stating that it causes cancer in lab rats. Then came Aspartame, truly an abomination.

Aspartame was first approved by the FDA in 1974. However, that approval was rescinded because laboratory studies showed it caused brain tumors. Even though these studies were never shown to be incorrect, in 1981 the FDA again approved Aspartame for some uses. Then in 1983 Aspartame was approved for use in soft drinks. More recently Aspartame was even approved for baked goods, which is really scary because of what happens to Aspartame when it is heated.

In every year since its approval, Aspartame has been the subject of 75 to 80% of the non-drug complaints received by the FDA. We're talking close to 10,000 cases. The cause of most adverse reactions are hard to pinpoint. They go unrecognized and unreported. According to the National Cancer Institute there has been a huge jump in the incidence of brain tumors in the '80's. Using 1983 as a baseline, in 1987 the estimated annual percentage change in brain tumors rose from 2.1% to 8.1% in males, and from 2.1% to 11.7% in females.

Every year since its approval, Aspartame has been the subject of 75% to 80% of the non-drug complaints received by the FDA.

By 1989 MIT researchers had surveyed more than 80 people who had suffered Aspartame induced brain seizures. The Community Nutrition Institute at MIT said, "The existence of these 80 cases meets the FDA's own definition of an imminent hazard to public health, which requires the FDA to expeditiously remove a product from the market." Of course, that hasn't happened.

There are three components to the Aspartame molecule, aspartic acid, phenylalanine and methanol. Methanol, or methyl alcohol or wood alcohol, is the stuff that has blinded and killed thousands of skid row drunks. As methanol breaks down in your body it forms formaldehyde and formic acid. Formaldehyde is a deadly neurotoxin—it's embalming fluid—it's a class A carcinogen. Formic acid is ant-sting poison. How would you like a fire ant bite to your brain? The absorption of methanol is greatly quickened by heating the Aspartame like in hot drinks or baked goods. Also, Aspartame decomposes during storage.

Aspartame is bad for everyone especially pilots and pregnant women. This poison is directly passed on to the developing fetus. Aspartame causes many symptoms. Here are a few:

Insomnia	**Loss of taste**	**Heart palpitations**
Fatigue	**Slurred speech**	**Blurred vision**
Breathing difficulty	**Ringing in ears**	**Rashes**
Anxiety attacks	**Muscle spasms**	**Hearing loss**

Blindness	**Numbness**	**Depression**
Headaches	**Memory loss**	**Nausea**
Seizures	**Dizziness**	**Death**

Oh, by the way, Aspartame also causes weight gain! That's right! It affects our hunger by causing cravings while storing the poisons in our fat cells so it's much harder to get rid of!

The commercial names of Aspartame are NutraSweet® and Equal®. There is, however, nothing nutritious about Aspartame. It is an artificial sweetener that is harmful to people. It's in thousands of products, even children's vitamins.

Don't you wish there was a sweetener that tasted good, was proven safe and had zero calories?

We have barely brushed the surface of this subject. If you want to learn more, consider these books: *The Deadly Deception*, *Bittersweet Aspartame*, *Sweetener Dearest and Aspartame, Is It Safe?*. You can also write to:

Aspartame Consumer Safety Network

P.O. Box 780634

Dallas, Texas 75378

or:

NutriVoice

P.O. Box 946

Oak Park, IL. 60303

Don't you wish there was a sweetener that tasted good and was good for us?...a sweetener proven safe, with no harmful side effects?...a sweetener that was not only safe but had great nutritional value as well?...a sweetener that did not contribute to any disease but actually helped get rid of some disease...a sweetener that tasted great but had ZERO calories? If we could find a sweetener like that, wouldn't it be welcomed with open arms? Wouldn't it be not only approved but promoted by our government?

There is a sweetener just like that! It's name is stevia. Our government could have promoted stevia but instead they banned it! Once again your health and the health of your children has been subordinated to the profits of agribusiness, drug companies, etc. For over ten years now while the FDA has banned stevia as a sweetener in the US, "Big Sugar Growers" have received enormous subsidies from the Department of Agriculture. At the same time the FDA was banning stevia it was approving Aspartame.

At the same time the FDA was banning stevia, it was approving Aspartame.

In 1976 an Illinois company was formed to explore the potential of stevia. By the early '80's stevia was being used in several food products like herbal teas. Sunrider International, a herb food company, was selling it as a sweetener called Tru-sweet®. In 1986 the FDA put a stop to all that. It told Sunrider it couldn't sell Tru-sweet. The FDA even went into Celestial Seasonings' (The herbal tea company) plant and warehouse and seized their entire stock of stevia. No legal reason was given for the seizure. It wasn't until 1991 that the FDA officially banned stevia, claiming that it was an "unsafe food additive."

Is Stevia Safe?

Japan has been researching and using stevia for 50 years. In the 1970's Japan declared stevia to be safe and nutritious and has been using it in all kinds of products like candy, ice cream, soft drinks, pickles, cookies, chewing gum, etc. Stevia has over 40% of the sweetener market in Japan, with not one single adverse effect reported in all those years.

The people of Paraguay have been using stevia during all of recorded history. Many other countries use stevia; Taiwan, Brazil, Korea, Thailand and China, to name just a few. However, as defined by the FDA, food additives are automatically considered unsafe until proven safe by domestic toxicity research.

This puts a tremendous burden on natural botanical products. You can't patent a banana, or any plant or animal. So it is very unusual for a company to spend the enormous amount of time, effort and money to do the toxicity research and submit it to the FDA. But, that is exactly what Sunrider International did in this case. (See Stevia article in Veggie Life, July, 1996). In fact, Sunrider submitted about 4,000 documents to the FDA. Finally, in September of 1995 the FDA approved stevia as a safe dietary supplement, but not as a sweetener or as a flavor enhancer.

A large number of companies have taken advantage of the ban lifting and are selling a stevia product. However, not all stevia is created equal. The genus stevia has more than 200 known species. Apparently, the best stevia for taste and nutritional value only grows in the subalpine highlands and mountainous countryside of Paraguay.

Stevia is said to help stabilize blood sugar levels, inhibit tooth decay and gum disease and soften the skin while healing blemishes and scarring.

Besides tasting good, having NO calories, and NO harmful side effects, traditionally stevia is said to help stabilize blood sugar levels, inhibit tooth decay and gum disease and soften the skin while healing blemishes and scarring. Stevia appears to contain anti-bacterial agents. Recent scientific research confirms the traditional good effects and adds others. Stevia extract, but not stevioside, stabilizes blood sugar levels. Stevioside is that part of stevia that tastes sweet. It is a sweet tasting isolate (300 times sweeter than sugar) with no harmful side effects but with no good nutritional effects either. Other studies show that stevia lowers elevated blood pressure but does not seem to effect normal blood pressure.

At least now you have a choice. You can choose sugar, you can choose artificial sweeteners or you can choose stevia. It's extremely easy to choose sugar and Aspartame because they are generally accepted and are in practically all of our foods. It's much harder to choose stevia simply because you first must avoid the other two. It can be done! It's worth the effort!

WORDS TO KNOW

Saccharides
Carbohydrates
Sucrose
Glucose
Endorphins
Opiates
Ritalin
Formaldehyde
Formic Acid
Methanol
Stevioside

SUMMARY

1. The average American eats 1,000 calories worth of sugar every day.
2. Sugar uses up many nutrients in the body like Vitamin B1, Calcium and Chromium.
3. Sugar causes neurological imbalances and behavioral problems.
4. About 80% of the food complaints received by the FDA are about Aspartame.
5. About 10% of Aspartame is methanol.
6. Methanol turns into formaldehyde and formic acid.
7. Formaldehyde is a deadly neurotoxin, formic acid is ant sting poison.
8. Pregnant women and pilots should never eat Aspartame.
9. Stevia is a safe, natural, calorie free, nutritious, sweet tasting herb.
10. The FDA banned stevia for years and still has not approved it as a sweetener
11. Stevia is also antibiotical and great for skin care

11

AMERICA'S MOST POPULAR BEVERAGES

Think about it for a minute. What do you think are the most popular beverages in the US? Most peoples' lists would include COFFEE, COLA, SODA, TEA, BEER, WINE, MILK and JUICE. Wait a minute. A few of you might have included WATER. Congratulations! But what kind of water do we drink? Let's take a real quick look at each beverage from a nutritional point of view.

1 PETER 2:11

Dear Friends, I urge you, as aliens and strangers in the world, to abstain from sinful desires, which war against your soul.

COFFEE

The most renowned ingredient in coffee, of course, is that powerful stimulant ... caffeine. It's the main reason we drink coffee—for the lift—or kick—it gives us. It's what gets our heart pumping and our adrenals producing. Yeah, I know, it also smells good when it is brewing. How about nutrition? Does coffee have any? NO! Sorry, but coffee contributes absolutely nothing positive to human body chemistry.

However, there have been copious numbers of studies that link caffeine to many diseases.

- Cancer—ovarian, bladder, pancreatic, renal, pelvic, etc.
- Fibrocystic breast and uterine disease.
- Spontaneous abortion, still birth, premature birth.

- High blood pressure, heart attack, stroke.
- Increased fat retention, increased cholesterol.

Coffee can harm your liver, kidneys, bladder, heart, stomach, bones, teeth and skin. Caffeine also depletes major nutrients, including calcium, zinc, copper, vitamins C, B5, B6 and the amino acid tyrosine. Caffeine inhibits digestion, particularly of carbohydrate.

Coffee can harm your liver, kidneys, bladder, heart, stomach, bones, teeth and skin.

Perhaps the most common problem caused by long term coffee consumption is its effect on the adrenal glands. Caffeine stimulates the production of noradrenalin, adrenalin and steroids. Over time this stimulation will cause the adrenal glands to become "washed out". Mental and emotional stress also contribute to this situation. The end result is low energy levels and blood sugar level irregularities.

Well, you say, you drink decaffeinated coffee. That might not be any safer. Most caffeine is removed by using a chemical solvent called methylene chloride. This chemical breaks down into formaldehyde and methanol, both of which are deadly neurotoxins and both are carcinogenic. Even if you got rid of the caffeine safely, there would still be 29 different acids, a large number of tars and zero nutrients. Coffee is a diuretic. That means it causes you to lose more water than you gain. Juan Valdez may be real cute in the commercials we see on television, but he is not doing us any favors.

TEA

Tea and cocoa also contain large amounts of caffeine, so everything we said about coffee would apply. However, the caffeine concentration is somewhat less, and cocoa and tea do have a few nutrients. So the overall effect is not as bad as coffee, but still not good for daily, long term consumption.

COLA & SODA

Soft drinks as a whole, are virtually nutrition free. Most contain four major substances; caffeine, sugar or Aspartame and carbon dioxide. We have just discussed caffeine. Sugar and Aspartame are major topics in the previous chapter. That leaves carbon dioxide. Carbon dioxide is what is used to give the soft drink its fizz or bubbles. While carbon dioxide is not a poison and is not normally considered dangerous, think about this. As our body burns food to make energy, the end products of the energy production process is water and carbon dioxide. The water can be used by our body but the carbon dioxide is a waste product and must be eliminated. Does it make sense to eat a lot of something that is a waste product to our body?

Does it make sense to eat a lot of something that is a waste product to our body?

Perhaps the worst thing about soft drinks is the large amount many people drink. They are popular with most Americans, particularly our youth. Can you believe the size of those jumbo drinks sold in convenience stores? 32 oz! 44 oz! Amazing, when you consider that just a 12 ounce can contains 10 teaspoons of sugar. Carbonated water, sugar, caffeine, artificial coloring, 240 calories per 12 ounces and zero nutrition—what a great drink, huh?

BEER, WINE & MIXED DRINKS (LIQUOR)

The main ingredient in all alcoholic beverages is ethanol. Ethanol is the substance that causes most of the changes in our body when we drink. One gram of alcohol contains seven calories. That means that one ounce of alcohol has 200 calories. Unfortunately, alcoholic calories cannot be converted to energy in our bodies. The metabolism of ethanol takes place exclusively in the liver. Actually, the process of breaking down alcohol is detoxing, not digestion. When a person drinks faster than his liver can detox the alcohol, he suffers from alcohol poisoning. The maximum alcohol detoxing capacity of a well-functioning liver is about one ounce per hour. That means, of course, that most drinkers suffer from alcohol poisoning.

Ethanol is a central nervous system depressant. Therefore, alcohol adversely affects nearly every part of our body—muscles, skin, infections, water balance, respiration, circulation, blood, motor performance, perception, reaction time, sleep, etc. Let's use one simple example. Alcohol depresses respiration, this in turn decreases the cough reflex, this slows down mucous transport, this allows germs to accumulate and proliferate, thus increasing the risk of pulmonary infection.

Alcohol weakens or damages the liver, pancreas, intestine, brain, adrenal glands and many other tissue groups. Hypoglycemia is very common among people who drink. Alcohol disrupts the blood sugar level and consistent drinking sets up a roller coaster effect in which the blood sugar first goes way up then drops like a rock.

For the alcoholic, those persons susceptible to alcohol, drinking can literally ruin their life. For those others who choose to drink, it is one more thing that leads to malnutrition. Ethanol consumption interferes with nutrient absorption and nutrient activation in the liver. It also causes a great number of free radicals. The micronutrients most often compromised are Folic Acid, Thiamin (B1), Pyridoxine (B6), Vitamin C, Vitamin A, Vitamin D, Vitamin B12, Calcium, Magnesium and Zinc.

Another mineral that is effected is Iron. Unlike the other nutrients, iron absorption increases with the ingestion of alcohol. That is why red wine is considered a blood builder. Red wine has both iron and alcohol. More iron can be either good or bad, depending on an individual's situation. Remember, iron overload is a significant problem in the U.S.

MILK

I know what you are thinking. If I tell you that milk is no good, I might as well attack patriotism and motherhood, too. I'll walk very softly and say that some milk is better than others, and milk used to be better than it is now. Fresh, raw goat's milk is pretty good food, but processed cow's milk is not good. Some authorities call it poison.

Everyone knows that milk is a major source of calcium and that we need lots of calcium. That's true enough. In fact, there are about 500 milligrams of calcium in every pint of milk. Unfortunately, when milk is pasteurized, it changes the molecular bonding of calcium in milk which makes it very difficult for our bodies to digest and utilize. Also, it is universal practice to add synthetic Vitamin D hormone to milk. As you may remember from an earlier discussion, we should not eat supplemental Vitamin D.

When milk is pasteurized, it changes the molecular bonding of calcium which makes it very difficult for our bodies to digest and utilize.

Milk is very high in fat and high in protein, two things we get too much of already. Milk causes excess mucous production and contributes to constipation for most people. Three quarters of the world's adult population lose their ability to digest milk, causing major digestive upset. There is an enzyme in homogenized milk called xanthine oxidase. Studies have shown this enzyme to promote free radical pathology.

Recently, the FDA approved a genetically engineered milk hormone called rBST, under extremely controversial circumstances! rBST (re-combinant Bovine Somatotiopin) forces cows to produce much more milk. It also causes more bacteria and puss, and therefore, more antibiotics in milk. During testing, rBST caused cancer in lab animals.

Several years ago the U.S. Congress passed a law prohibiting the FDA from approving any drug that caused cancer in lab animals. This law is known as the Delaney Amendment. In order to approve rBST the FDA had to first minimize their interpretation of the Delaney Amendment, which they did. The story of rBST and other Dairy Industry efforts reads like an espionage novel, with the American public as the victim.

If you drink milk or eat cheese and other dairy products, do yourself and your family a huge favor. Read the new book by Robert Cohen, *MILK: The Deadly Poison*, (ISBN #0-9659-196-0-9). Get the truth, then as always, decide for yourself!

FRUIT JUICES

Fruit juices should be great beverages although they are pretty concentrated. You might want to mix them with distilled water, say at a 50-50 ratio. This would apply more to non-citrus juices.

There are really only two major problems with fruit juice. First, most juice commercially available is processed, made from concentrate and pasteurized, thereby removing or destroying much of their nutritional content. Secondly, residues from pesticides, fungicides and herbicides have been found in alarming amounts in many juices. For example, some juices contain over 6 mg. of fluoride per liter.

Some juices contain over 6 mg. of fluoride per liter.

WATER

We devoted an entire chapter to water. You might want to review it at this time. (Chapter 15)

In my opinion, the perfect beverage for our waste laden and fast-paced world would be concentrated whole food nutrition dissolved in steam distilled water and consumed regularly throughout the day.

WORDS TO KNOW

Ethanol

SUMMARY

1. Coffee is loaded with caffeine, tars and acids but contains NO NUTRIENTS at all.
2. Coffee contributes to a great number of diseases.
3. Tea and cocoa are almost as bad as coffee.
4. Alcohol is not digested—it is detoxified in the liver.
5. Alcohol contributes to a large variety of problems in our health and in our life.
6. Processed milk is not a very good beverage.
7. Many fruit juices have been contaminated with chemicals from pesticides, fungicides, herbicides, etc.

12

STRESS

Without stress no living system can function. It helps bring about that balance in the body we call homeostasis. The stress function in our bodies is God created and good. Without it we would be in big trouble. It's the fact that we don't handle stress properly that hurts us.

In our modern society there are three stages of stress that a person goes through. First is recognition. That is simply knowing that we are in a stressful situation. Then comes adaptation (some authorities call this stage resistance) where our mind and body "handle" the stress. If it is handled properly, the stress will be used for its intended purpose and will dissipate, causing no harmful effects. If the stress is not handled properly, it brings on the third stage which is called fatigue.

Stressors occur both outside our body and inside our body. Recognition of outside stress comes through our nervous system and through our five senses; sight, hearing, smell, touch and taste. They tell us about our environment and go through that portion of our brain called the thalamus. Information from inside our body goes to the hypothalamus which controls automatic and semi-automatic functions like sleep, hunger, heart rate, etc.

The thalamus and hypothalamus must communicate constantly or we lose homeostasis. A simple

PHILIPPIANS 4:6

Do not be anxious about anything, but in everything, by prayer and petition, with thanksgiving, present your requests to God.

example would be going into a walk-in freezer. The brain receives a lot of information very quickly, probably the most important is that it is cold in here. The body starts doing things to conserve heat and make more heat. It stops perspiration, closes skin pores (sometimes we see the result as goose bumps), routes blood away from the skin, converts glycogen into glucose to be burned, and many other things.

When we relive an event in our mind, the stress reaction in our bodies is the same as when the actual experience happened.

The amazing fact is that in the average second our brain stem is bombarded by 100 million impulses from our inside environment and our outside environment. Fortunately, there are many filters and suppressors that handle most impulses before they reach the brain. Only a few hundred impulses are actually processed by our brain every second. ...ONLY! One thing that helps reduce brain processing is memory. Once we have stored a particular solution to a problem, we don't have to solve it again and again. We simply play back the tape from stored memory. So the impulses we notice are new or life threatening. Have you ever gone to visit someone who lives very close to a railroad track? In the middle of the night the train goes speeding by, you wake up thinking the world is coming to an end, but the people who live there sleep right through it? Their filters and suppressors protect them from those impulses.

The thalamus and hypothalamus are sub-cortical or sub-cortex. These parts of our brain are developed and functioning at birth. The cortex of the brain is undeveloped when we are born, and grows throughout our life. So the cortex is where things are stored—memory. As a matter of fact, every memory is stored there—nothing is lost! The first time we have an experience we are emotionless about it because emotion only comes with experience. When we experience something, we receive it into our thalamus and/or hypothalamus which is protected by filters and suppressors. But when we recall that event from memory, it comes from the cortex which does not have any filters to protect us. When we relive an event in our mind, the stress reaction in our bodies is exactly the same type as the actual experience, even though it may not be as strong. In other words, recalling something causes the same chemical, biochemical and physiological reaction in our bodies as the event itself. Not only are we unprotected from memories, but, if the event was unpleasant, the memory is now mixed with a negative emotion like fear or anger.

The end result of recalling negative events is to place our body in that third stress stage of fatigue.

The major chemical reaction to a stressful stimulus is called the fight or flight syndrome. This is where the body is prepared to either run away from danger or stand and fight it. Let's use an example. Let's say that it is dinner time and just before you sit down to eat you let the dog outside. About ten minutes later, when you are half way through your meal, you hear a terrible squeal of tires on the street in front of the house. Instantly, many chemical and physical changes occur in your body. Digestion stops, hydrochloric acid production stops, adrenalin and cordicoids are produced, blood is channeled away from the stomach and skin to the muscles, glycogen is changed into glucose, and scores of other changes take place. You jump up and run outside, afraid you will find Rover smashed in the street. Fortunately, the noise happened just down the block. No one was hurt and there is Rover sitting on the front porch, no damage done. You pick him up, take him in the house and breathe a prayer of thanks. You wait for your heart to stop racing. It takes a few minutes to come back to normal and you resume your meal. Notice that you did physical things to use up the physical chemicals that were produced. However, when we replay an event in our mind, particularly one that didn't have a happy ending, the same chemicals are made by our body, but they are usually not used up. When these chemicals are not used up, they cause changes in our body that we call tension, nervousness, anxiety, depression, etc. So the end result of recalling negative events is to place our body in that third stress stage of fatigue.

But let's say you are constantly irritated or depressed on the job or by a particular situation you find yourself in. It doesn't really matter what the stimulus is what the stress is. It causes the same reaction in the body. Hydrochloric acid production is stopped, the blood bypasses the liver and goes to the muscles to give the strength to either fight or run. Let's say the stress situation continues to the point that you worry that it is going to reoccur. Worrying about the situation causes the same physiological and biochemical changes to happen as the actual event. It is interesting that this only happens to man; apparently animals don't worry, only man worries.

After a while of this stress and worry over stress, the body moves into the fatigue stage, and it begins to malfunction and become out of balance. So in our present example, the hydrochloric acid production goes up, and it goes up at the wrong time; at the time when the stomach is empty. Now hydrochloric acid is not discriminating. It doesn't know the difference between food protein and stomach lining protein. It only knows how to break down protein. So we get an ulcer. Your body was not designed to be sick! The only reason why people get sick is because cells can't function properly. The cause can be either physical or psychological, an event or a thought, a nutritional deficiency or toxic waste, bad timing or imbalance. Every cell needs proper nutrition, proper cleanliness and proper timing for communication with the rest of the body.

Stress that happens here and now will never make you sick! It is always the emotion attached to the event from stored memory that makes us sick. FEAR is the most destructive emotion.

Never put a negative emotion caused from an event or circumstance into your subconscious—always deal with it here and now. If you don't, it will come back as tension, headache, tight shoulders, constipation—something. The Bible says in Proverbs 14:30, "A heart at peace gives life to the body, but envy rots the bones." Ephesians 4:26 is good advice, "In your anger do not sin. Do not let the sun go down while you are still angry." This would probably apply to other negative emotions as well.

Many headaches are caused by situations in life that cause you to get tense. When the headache comes, you recognize the discomfort. Someone, at sometime, probably told you it was a migraine. This sets up in your memory what a migraine headache is. As we remember the discomforts of a migraine, it brings on fear and worry that we will get another one sometime. So at the first signs of a headache the memory of it kicks in the fear and worry which in turn, so often, will produce the headache. In other words, your mind is trying its dead level best to produce what you fear will happen. I've even heard people say, "I'm getting another headache and it's going to be a bad one." Or "I'm getting another infection and it's a bad one, I just know it." And all too often they are right.

What do you do about it? Just be a little smarter than your mind. Your mind will work on whatever thoughts you place in it. Proverbs 23:7 says, "for as he thinketh in his heart, so is he." and Proverbs 17:1, "Better a dry crust with peace and quiet than a house full of feasting with strife."

We have been talking about our nervous system, our sensory system and the stimuli they work on. Any time your mind receives a stimulus you will get a total body response to that stimulus. If you don't like the response you are getting, change the stimulus! For example, when you feel yourself becoming tense, don't think about a headache, practice a relaxation technique. If the tension is caused by an event, handle it right now. If your boss has made you mad again, talk to him, or pray and give it to the Lord, but don't harbor that anger or other negative emotion overnight, because if you do, you have just stored it in your memory to come back as some illness or disease. And above all, don't replay the event over and over in your mind; forgive your boss, not so much for his sake but for yours! If you don't like the response, change the stimulus. Remember, fear can drive us into anxiety or depression. So don't worry about things, handle them right away. Then you will turn stress into success. That's the way God intended it to work. As Christians we have God's promise on it; Romans 8:28, "And we know that all things work together for good to them that love God, to them who are called according to His purpose."

Our body reacts the same to an event or a replay of the event from memory.

It's not always bad to find ourselves in unpleasant circumstances and situations. It is there that we gain wisdom. It is there that we perfect our character. The only reason we stay in that unpleasant situation is, because we haven't learned to change the stimulus that brings on that response. Man might be the only creature that does the same thing day after day and still expects a different response. Bacteria don't like the response caused by antibiotics so they change. Insects don't like the effect of insecticides so they change, they don't just worry about getting sprayed again. Test animals stop doing the things that cause an electric shock. But man, who doesn't like the effects of worry, worries about it, and even fears it. So it doesn't matter whether the feared event happens or not, because the fear and worry bring on all of the same negative physiological things that the event did. Our body reacts the same to an event or a replay of the event from memory. So many people go through life in the valleys with stress as an enemy, rather than using stress as an instructor and therefore a very positive and natural and beneficial force.

When you are in a stressful situation, there are a couple of kinds of hormones that are secreted into the bloodstream. One is called glucocordicoid. These are the cordicoids that promote glucose metabolism. Another group is called anti-inflammatory cordicoids, like cortisone which stops inflammation. Another group is called mineral cordicoids and they promote inflammation. After a stressful event the liver is supposed to bring all these different cordicoids back into balance. When the stress is real, that is, the event actually happenes, we get up, move around, run, fight or whatever. That physical activity allows the liver to perform its balancing job after the event. However, when the stressful event is replayed from memory, all the chemicals are made, but not used, and the liver is bypassed and does not balance them out.

So the mineral cordicoids stay high and when they pass through the kidneys, they can damage the tiny tubular structure and cause hypertension—high blood pressure. These mineral cordicoids have an affinity for our joints so they can get deposited there. Since they are pro-inflammatory, they bring on an inflammation in our joints that we call arthritis. Now this is not the only imbalance that can contribute to hypertension, arthritis and other diseases, but it is one of them.

Knowledge is the number one enemy of fear!

Sometimes the fear of something is worse for you than if whatever you fear actually happens to you. In order to get rid of the fear you must be able to accept the worst consequences of it, after you have learned everything about it. For example, if you fear cancer, learn all you can about cancer, the effective habits and lifestyles that prevent cancer development. Read the stories about people who have cured themselves of cancer. The more you know about something the less fearful it becomes. Knowledge is the number one enemy of fear!

Nearly everyone will improve their health if they stop doing the things that make them sick. The blueprint of a perfect body is still there in every cell. It's called DNA and RNA. Lifestyle changes are needed and that's very difficult for most of us, because we do the things we like to do until they become a habit. To break a habit takes conscious effort and discipline, and many of us are unwilling to apply the self-discipline necessary to make the change. For those that will, spiritual, mental and physical health is the reward, and it's well worth the effort.

WORDS TO KNOW

Thalamus

Hypothalamus

Cortex

Stimulus

Corticoids

SUMMARY

1. Stress is normal, natural and should be good for us.
2. Our bodies produce certain chemicals every time we are stressed.
3. Handle a stressful event right away.
4. Don't "replay" a stressful event over and over in your mind.
5. Don't 'worry' about things—take steps to be in control.
6. Always forgive people, for their sake, but mostly for your own.
7. You will improve your health when you stop doing the things that make you sick.

13

GOD'S DIETARY SUGGESTIONS

Because for so many hundreds of years, men without spiritual comprehension have been exalted as authorities, their lack of wisdom has become paramount in their teachings that are passed on generation to generation. As each new generation of "teachers" adds their "light", the drift away from the original truth and their meanings is often incomprehensible. It is for this reason that the Scriptures must be re-examined and looked upon as God's treasure and gift to mankind.

JAMES 1:22

Do not merely listen to the Word, and so deceive yourselves. Do what it says.

Man has written over 30 million laws and has not succeeded in improving upon the original commandments. Science has researched, examined, dissected, guessed and groped; medicine has poked, prodded, cut, injected, rejected, mutilated, experimented and defiled in the name of progress, and in essence has begun to find that the 3500 year old hygienic and dietary laws written down by Moses are absolute and infallible after all. In spite of this, most Christians still ignore the knowledge that is so freely given to whomsoever will receive.

In order to talk about unclean food we first must take a look at the Old Testament law and our attitude toward it.

The laws of God recorded in the Scriptures can generally be classified into three categories: 1) the moral law, 2) the dietary law and 3) the ceremonial law. Man, being imperfect and unrighteous cannot keep the law. Herein lies the Good News: Christ kept all of the moral law, the dietary law and He was the fulfillment of the ceremonial law. Now all of His righteousness is charged to our account, because we receive Him as our Messiah-Redeemer, as our substitute who paid the death penalty for our transgressions.

The Scriptures must be re-examined and looked upon as God's treasure and gift to mankind.

"There is, therefore, now no condemnation to those which are in Christ Jesus ... for the law of the Spirit of life in Christ Jesus hath made me free from the law of sin and death - for what the law could not do through physical weakness ... God sending His own Son in the likeness of sinful flesh, and for sin, condemned sin in the flesh that the righteousness of the law might be fulfilled in us who walk not after the flesh but after the Spirit." (Romans 8:1-4).

As far as salvation and eternal life are concerned, the believer is not to be in bondage under the law. Christ paid the penalty of our violation (Galatians 3:10-13). Christ died our death and bore away our eternal punishment. We now are dead, legally, before God through Christ's death—but also eternally alive through His resurrection (Romans 6:11).

"We groan within ourselves, waiting for ... the redemption of our body" (Romans 8:23). As long as we live in this body, we must realize that it is subject to all the physical laws that God laid down for its normal function and well-being. When this body shall be changed and "fashioned like unto His glorious body" (Philippians 3:21) and at His appearance when "we shall be like Him" (I John 3:2) we can then forget all these laws that God made for our physical welfare in this present world.

So there is no legalism in trying to keep the law, but only a desire to please Him. "Don't you know that you yourselves are God's temple and that God's Spirit lives in you? If anyone destroys God's temple, God will destroy him; for God's temple is sacred, and you are that temple." (I Corinthians 3:16-17).

Most people think it is wrong to kill or steal or commit adultery; that is, they accept the moral law, but those same people reject the dietary law. On what grounds? There is none! God's laws are still in effect regarding this earthly life. Jesus said "...and the Scripture cannot be broken..." (John 10:35) we merely break ourselves over it, read Deuteronomy, Chapter 28.

We don't really break God's laws, we merely break ourselves over it.

God's dietary suggestions are really very simple. We are to eat fresh vegetables, fruits, seeds, grains and nuts (Genesis 1:29). Then He added bulbs, roots and herbs (Genesis 3:18). After the flood, meat was added to man's diet (Genesis 9:3), "but you must not eat meat that has its lifeblood still in it" (Genesis 9:4). When God gave Moses and the Israelites the Law, He further restricted our diets by telling us that fat was NEVER to be eaten (Leviticus 3:17). He also differentiated between the meat that is good for us and the meat that would make us sick (Leviticus, Chapter 11 and Deuteronomy, Chapter 14).

CLEAN AND UNCLEAN MEATS

Red Meats:

Clean: beef, lamb, mutton, veal

Unclean: pork, dog, horse, mule

Game:

Clean: buffalo, caribou, deer, elk, moose

Unclean: armadillo, bear, beaver, muskrat, opossum, rabbit, raccoon, squirrel, wild boar, woodchuck

Poultry & Game Birds:

Clean: capon, chicken, Cornish hen, dove, grouse, guinea fowl, lark, partridge, pheasant, pigeon, quail, snipe, turkey

Unclean: duck, eagle, falcon, goose, osprey

Sea Fish:

Clean: bass, bluefish, butterfish, cod, croaker, cusk, flounder, grouper, haddock, hake, halibut, herring, kipper, mullet, pilchard, pollock, pompano, porgy, red snapper, rose fish, salmon, sardine, sea trout, shad, sole, whiting

Unclean: blue marlin, eel, lamprey, mackerel, octopus, squid, swordfish, tuna, turbot, crab, lobster, shrimp, oyster, scallops, prawns

Modern science is beginning to understand why the Scripturally "unclean" foods are bad for us.

It appears that we should not eat milk and meat at the same meal (Exodus 23:19), and finally, the Holy Spirit tells us not to eat food sacrificed to idols, blood, and the meat of strangled animals (Acts 15:28-29).

Most of us don't have a big problem not eating the meat of dogs or horses or rats. When was the last time you had a rat sandwich? But when was the last time you had a ham sandwich? Both rats and pigs are an abomination to God (Isaiah 66:17).

Modern science is beginning to understand why the Scripturally "unclean" foods are bad for us. The Bible says don't eat fat. Why? Fatty protein molecules in the blood stream are deposited on the inner wall of our arteries. As it piles up it narrows and irritates the vessels, encouraging more formation of such deposits (see Chapters 1 & 6). It isn't long before the blood does not have sufficient room to flow freely, causing high blood pressure, blood clots, heart attacks, strokes and other degenerative diseases. The Bible says don't eat blood. Why not? If we liken the blood vessels to a railroad transportation system, then the blood would be the railroad cars. Most everything that needs to move throughout the body uses this transportation system; oxygen, nutrients, enzymes, hormones, toxins, poisons, viruses, germs, waste products and many other things both good and bad. Most of the bad things are cleaned out of the blood by the liver and kidneys. These toxins, poisons, waste products, etc. are stored in the bladder then eliminated from the body as urine. In other words, just prior to being urine, it was in the blood.

Other than fat and blood, our biggest problems are probably with pork and shellfish. Let's consider the swine. Pigs will eat anything! That's why they were created, to be a scavenger. An animal will die, lie in the sun and bloat, become full of maggots and rot and a pig will eat up all this filth. It will eat its own young, garbage, the feces of other animals...anything!! Because of the hog's anatomy (a single stomach arrangement) his putrid and polluted swill becomes flesh on its bones in just four hours. In contrast, clean animals (sheep, ox, cow, etc.) have three stomachs to clean and refine its fresh grass and grain diet. It takes about 24 hours to make meat on its bones.

Other than fat and blood, our biggest problems are probably with pork and shellfish.

You might think that if a pig were raised in a clean environment and fed only wholesome food, it then would be good to eat. That's simply not true. The fat and lean are together in the swine, whereas in clean animals such as beef, they are marbled. Swine flesh rots from the inside out—beef from the outside. Because of its very nature, unclean meat burns up too fast in our digestive systems and causes a net loss of energy. In other words, the human body uses more energy to get rid of it than it gives in return.

All shellfish are either filter feeders or bottom feeders. They perform the same function as the hog-scavengers. They are very high in many toxic chemicals and metals, like mercury poisoning. From time to time you have probably seen the warnings; don't eat the scallops or oysters because of the high bacteria. If you like Escargot ask yourself this question. How does a snail go to the bathroom?

Many more things could be said on the subject but perhaps Paul sums it up best in I Corinthians 6:19-20, "What? Know ye not that your body is the temple of the Holy Spirit who is in you, Whom ye have of God, and; ye are not your own? For ye are bought with a price; therefore, glorify God in your body and in your spirit, which are God's."

Another very large problem with eating swine flesh is parasites. We can get at least 18 different kinds of worms, from the simple intestinal parasite to the deadly trichinella spiralis. Parasites are one of the world's leading causes of death. They don't kill us too often in this country, but they are still a big problem. For example, it is estimated that more than half of the people in Florida have parasites of some kind.

Another very large problem with eating swine flesh is parasites.

The most prevalent source of parasites is eating pork and the very worst parasite is trichinella spiralis, which we get exclusively from swine flesh. I also think you should know that there is no inspection for trichinae in any pork sold in the U.S. Dr. Laird S. Goldsborough writes, "a single serving of infected pork—even a single mouthful—can kill, cripple or condemn the victim to a lifetime of aches and pains." Senator Thomas C. Desmond, who served as chairman of the New York Trichinosis Commission stated, "Physicians have confused Trichinosis with some fifty ailments, ranging from typhoid fever to acute alcoholism. That pain in your arm or leg may be arthritis or rheumatism, but it may be trichinosis; that pain in your back may mean a gallbladder involvement, but it may mean trichinosis."

The trichinae is just one of eighteen worms found in the swine. There is a large round worm, the gullet worm, three kinds of stomach worms, a tiny hair worm, a hookworm and the thorn-headed worm, in the small intestines. There are several species of nodular worms and one species of whip worm in the colon, and the kidney worm. The large round worm can be as long as eighteen inches.

There are several other ways to get parasites. Blood-sucking insects introduce infective larva into the skin, and some larva invade exposed skin directly from the soil or grass, and we can get some from our pets. They can even come from fruits and vegetables that are not properly washed.

SUMMARY

1. The Bible contains "Laws" that can be divided into three general categories:
    - A) Moral Law
    - B) Dietary Law
    - C) Ceremonial Law
2. Jesus kept all the laws and fulfilled the ceremonial law.
3. Trying to live by scriptural suggestions is not being legalistic, its being obedient.
4. The physical laws that God created are still in effect—like the law of gravity.
5. God's dietary laws are not designed to limit our pleasures but to keep us healthy.

14

FASTING

In Western societies like the United States the outward manifestation of the power of God is rarely seen and even more rarely believed in. We have been raised from our youth to believe the precepts of secular humanism and the scientific method. While in more "primitive" cultures where the everyday lives of the people include the supernatural, God reveals Himself through mighty signs and wonders and miracles. It is very unfortunate that our belief (faith) has eroded to such an extent that we no longer seek to utilize that great power or to do the things necessary to make it real in our lives.

PROVERBS 13:19

A longing fulfilled is sweet to the soul, but fools detest turning from evil.

Remember the story in Mark, Chapter 9, of the boy who was possessed by a demon? Jesus was away praying and His disciples tried to cast the demon out but couldn't. Later, Jesus was asked why, and His reply can be found in Mark 9:29, "And He said unto them, This kind can come forth by nothing, but by prayer and fasting". Apparently there is power in prayer and fasting. Couple that with faith and you have the stuff that miracles are made of.

In recent years one of the largest Christian movements has been in Korea. Virtually every Christian church in Korea holds a prayer meeting every morning at 5:00 A.M., 365 days a year. When asked why they do this, their answers are short and direct: "Because that's where the power is!"

The Full Gospel Central Church of Seoul, Korea has bought a large plot of land just south of the demilitarized zone that they call Fasting Prayer Mountain. Founded in 1973, careful records are kept about all that happens there. The latest figures show over one million visitors a year. A commercial bus company has scheduled hourly runs over the forty-five minute route from Seoul. Many visitors go to attend the revival type services that are held, but over 100,000 individuals a year go specifically for prayer and fasting. A staff of no less than 130 full and part-time ministers are on duty to instruct them in the correct method of fasting for periods of from one to forty days. The only restaurant is a fasting withdrawal service with scientifically planned menus. About 500 private individual prayer grottos have been dug into the mountain itself, and every one is occupied almost twenty-four hours a day. The founder, Joshil Choi says, "With prayer and fasting we can cast Satan out, bring deliverance from bondage, and receive healing for our physical bodies." The official scriptural motto of Fasting Prayer Mountain comes from Isaiah 58:6: "Is this not the fast that I have chosen; to loose the bond of wickedness, to undo the heavy burdens, to let the oppressed go free, and that you break every yoke?"

The Bible is absolutely loaded with examples of fasting.

The Bible is absolutely loaded with examples of fasting—Old Testament, New Testament, even Jesus Himself fasted and taught us how to fast. Yet in America today, fasting is taught in less than 5% of our churches. Why?

Do you remember the story about Esther and Mordecai? Esther had won a beauty contest and had become a Queen of King Xerxes. The Jews, of course, had been conquered and scattered throughout the Medo Persian Empire. The story takes place in Susa. The villain is Haman, who is the highest noble, right under the King. Haman wants everyone to bow down to him, but Mordecai won't. Haman is furious and plots to kill, not only Mordecai, but every single Jew in the kingdom. Mordecai finds out about the plot and asks

Esther to go to King Xerxes to save her people. Esther would be risking her life if she approach the King in this way! So Esther calls a fast for every Jew in Susa. It was a total fast with no food and no water for three (3) days. All the Jews beg God's forgiveness and protection. God moves! The story ends with Haman being hung on the very gallows that he built to kill Mordecai. Mordecai gets Haman's entire estate, and Jews throughout the kingdom are victorious over their enemies. There is POWER in PRAYER and FASTING.

Perhaps the most informative scriptural passages on fasting are Isaiah 58:1-14 and Matthew 6:16-18. Please study them. There are so many others! I will list some of them for those who want to study further:

Zechariah 7:5
Psalm 69:10
Psalm 35:13
Joel 1:14
Joel 2:12
II Samuel 1:12
Luke 5:33-35
Daniel 6:18
II Samuel 12:16
Acts 13:3
II Corinthians 11:27
Acts 14:23
Ezra 8:23
Daniel 9:3
I Samuel 7:6
Nehemiah 9:1-2
Luke 2:37
Matthew 2:18
Deuteronomy 9:18
Nehemiah 1:4
Luke 18:12
Jeremiah 14:12
Matthew 4:2
Exodus 34:28
I Kings 21:12
I Kings 19:8
Judges 20:26
Jeremiah 36:9
I Samuel 31:13
Jonah 3:5-8
Acts 10:30
II Corinthians 6:5
Matthew 9:14

One of the most remarkable stories concerning

fasting happened not long ago (1953) to an American. There was a young man named Ken Cantrell who was in the U.S. Navy on board an aircraft carrier in the Mediterranean Sea. The Lord had called him to a 21 day water only fast. On the 17th day of that fast Ken Cantrell was at work in the catapult room just below the flight deck. About a dozen of his shipmates were also in that room when high octane aviation fuel spilled and exploded. All those men were instantly incinerated, all except Ken Cantrell. For the next hour or so, in full view of hundreds of other sailors, Ken Cantrell walked in and out of that inferno carrying the charred bodies of his friends. After the fire was under control the captain told Ken Cantrell to report to sick bay. As he walked down through the patients in sick bay, everyone of them was instantly healed. You can check it out yourself in the archives of the U.S. Navy. Doesn't this remind you of three young Jewish boys that were thrown into the fiery furnace many years ago? The same power that was active in the time of Daniel is just as active and just as powerful today.

Ken Cantrell walked in and out of that inferno carrying the charred bodies of his friends.

Jesus says in Matthew 6 that there is a reward for proper fasting. I don't know about you, but I like the idea of a reward from God. In Isaiah 58, it says that your healing will quickly appear during a proper fast. That could be an important promise for most of us.

So what is fasting anyway? Fasting is much more than simply not eating. Fasting is giving up something physical or carnal or worldly in order to separate yourself unto God. You can fast food or drink or cigarettes or sex or movies or anything and everything that has to do with the physical world while seeking the spiritual world.

A well-known Pastor tells of an experience he had on an airplane a couple of years ago. He was seated next to a man who was obviously in prayer. When the meal came the man declined even to take a beverage. The Pastor, noticing his prayerful attitude, told the man he was a Pastor and wanted to know if he could agree with him in prayer. The man said he didn't know. He said he was a Satanist fasting and praying for the destruction of Christian marriages. Fasting is giving up the physical while seeking the spiritual, and it's important to do it the right way.

The promise of quick healing during a fast might be the result of a process called autolysis. This is the process of cell replication and reproduction. Our bodies are made up of trillions of cells. Everyone of those cells wear out and must be replaced periodically. The main construction material for cells is amino acids or protein. During a fast the body does not receive protein from an external source (eating) so it procures the dynamic form amino acids from old cells that it tears apart. You might say the body recycles the protein. The great thing is that the body will go out and get the weakest, the dying, the sickest, the malignant cells and build brand new strong, healthy cells out of them. That's a good trade isn't it, the weakest cells for the strongest? Of course, when the body tears apart those sick cells, there are a lot of toxins and waste products released into the system. So, it's a real good idea to flush out the body by drinking a lot of pure water.

Jesus says in Matthew 6, that there is a reward for proper fasting.

That's why some people say they can't fast. They say it makes them sick, and that can be true unless it is done properly. Some things you might expect during a fast are; headache, bad breath, thick tongue, sticky teeth, dark, smelly urine, etc. as those waste products exit through the eliminating organs of the body.

Many people fast regularly. Once a week for 24 hours. Every three or four months an extended fast of from three to seven days. It sometimes is a water only fast, sometimes a juice fast and sometimes a cleansing fast. (Review Chapter 7, concerning detoxification)

WORDS TO KNOW

Autolysis

SUMMARY

1. Fasting is giving up something physical to become closer to the spiritual.
2. Fasting and prayer go together.
3. There are many, many examples of fasting and prayer in the Bible.
4. Jesus tells us there is a reward for proper fasting. (Matthew 6).
5. The Bible promises that healing will occur quickly during and after a proper fast. (Isaiah:58).
6. Improper fasting can make you sick.

15

WATER

Water...after oxygen, is the most essential nutrient in your life!!!

Vibrant health is a goal we all share.

PURE water more than any other substance will help you achieve it!

You might have heard that there is a shortage of water. That's not true! As a matter of fact, water is abundant and practically indestructible. There is approximately 326 million cubic miles of water on this planet. The same water cycles endlessly.

So what is all the hubbub about? It's the lack of PURE water that's the problem. You see, over 97% of water is in the oceans and seas (salt water), over 2% is in ice caps and glaciers (relatively unaccessible). Only six tenths of one percent (.6%) of the water is in lakes, rivers, ground water and the atmosphere. Even this small amount would be plenty if it were available where we needed it and if man hadn't ruined it. An article in a Tallahassee newspaper recently said, "the 'Good News' is that we must now drink recycled sewer water and the 'Bad News' is that there isn't enough of it!"

3 JOHN 2

Dear Friend, I pray that you may enjoy good health and that all may go well with you, even as your soul is getting along well.

Do you know how important water is to your life and health? Consider these facts about water in your body.

- An average person doing light work in a temperate climate loses about five pints of water a day, and must replace it.
- A man at rest is losing over half an ounce of water through his skin every hour.
- The maximum daily loss and replacement of water ever recorded is about 50 pints.
- Breathing, digestion, elimination, glandular activities, heat dissipation, secretion and many other body functions can only be performed in water solutions.
- The adult body should be about 70% water. A newborn baby is approximately 90% water.
- Percentage of water making up the human body; Brain 75% - Heart 75% - Muscle 75% - Lungs 86% - Liver 85% - Kidneys 83% - Bone 22% - Blood 83% - Saliva 95% - Fat 1%.
- The body uses only pure water. All impurities must be removed by the liver at great cost of energy. These impurities must be washed out of the body using...you guessed it...still more water, or it will be stored in our tissues.

Many of us are human, toxic waste dumps.

Many of us are human toxic waste dumps. None can deny, of course, that the body requires large quantities of water to thrive and survive. We will die without water in just a few days.

Many volumes have been written describing man's senseless pollution of our water supplies. You can refer to them for the gory details.

In the last 20 years or so we have tried to protect our environment somewhat. While we have succeeded in slowing down the rate of pollution, today our worldwide water supply is in the worst condition in history.

TAP WATER ALERT

Read today's top news stories for the real truth about your drinking water ...

"More than 1 in 5 Americans unknowingly drink tap water polluted with feces, radiation or other contaminants...Nearly 1,000 deaths each year and at least 400,000 cases of waterborne illness may be attributed to contaminated water..." The New York Times, June 2, 1995

"The parasite [cryptosporidium] that killed more than 100 people in Milwaukee two years ago has been found in drinking water systems that serve 45 million people..."Houston Chronicle, June 2, 1995

"Parasite in water is widespread...can be dangerous, even fatal, to people with weakened immune systems." USA TODAY, March 30, 1995

"Some individuals, federal officials said last week, should not drink water straight from the tap because a disease-causing parasite can slip right through many municipal water treatment systems." U.S. News & World Report, June 26, 1995

"Federal statutes do not require municipal water authorities to clean cryptosporidium from water reservoirs. Some lawmakers and industry lobbyists are also pushing for relaxation of the Safe Drinking Water Act." The Washington Post, June 2, 1995

There are over 20,000 toxic chemicals which are now present in America's water systems.

There are over 20,000 toxic chemicals which are now present in America's water systems, and about 500 new chemicals are introduced every year. Municipal water companies use many different chemicals to "clean up" the drinking water. For example:

Activated carbon
Activated silica
Aluminum ammonium sulfate
Aluminum chloride solution
Aluminum potassium sulfate
Aluminum sulfate
Alum liquid
Anhydrous, ammonia
Aqua, ammonia
Ammonium silicofluoride
Ammonium sulfate
Bentonite
Bromine
Calcium carbonate
Calcium hydroxide
Calcium hyposchlorite
Calcium oxide
Calcium dioxide
Chlorinated copperas
Chlorinated lime
Chlorine
Chlorine dioxide
Copper sulfate
Disodium phosphate
Dolomitic hydrated lime
Dolomitic lime
Ferric chloride
Ferric sulfate
Fluosilicic acid
Hydrofluoric acid
Ozone
Sodium aluminate
Sodium bicarbonate
Sodium bisulfite
Sodium carbonate
Sodium chloride
Sodium fluoride
Sodium hexametaphosphate
Sodium hyroxide
Sodium hypochlorite
Sodium silicate
Sodium sulfite
Sodium thiosulfate
Sulfur dioxide
Sulfuric acid
Tetrasodium pyrophosphate
Trisodium phosphate

When these "beneficial" chemicals are injected into our water supply, they mingle with chemicals already there. Just what combinations there are in our drinking water or what effect they might have on the human body is unknown.

There is one chemical that is present in virtually every water system - chlorine. But we need chlorine because it kills bacteria, right? Sure, but did you know that chlorine interacts with natural humus and Humic acid to form THM's (Trihalomethanes) which are carcinogens. Perhaps the best known THM is chloroform. Most water utilities seem unruffled by the fact that their standard operating procedure puts a cancer causing substance into every glass of tap water!

Most water utilities seem unruffled by the fact that their standard operating procedure puts a cancer causing substance into every glass of tap water.

And then, of course, there is fluoride - truly an abomination! It is one of the most deadly poisons known to man, and a toxic waste from the smelting industries and phosphate fertilizer production plants that is being disposed of in our water. See Chapter 9.

We will drink it, pure or not. That two or three quarts of water we drink every day is not optional! We humans will drink any water available when our bodies demand water to save us from dehydration and death. The only question is what kind of water will we drink, coffee, soda, beer, tap water, bottled water or pure water? The choice of beverages is almost endless, but remember, the body uses pure water and must purify nearly everything except already pure water.

We need to realize that contaminants and toxic chemicals, introduced into our body through our drinking water, interfere with normal metabolic and enzymatic activities, while creating copious numbers of free radicals. We can understand this better when we consider that when our body makes chemicals like enzymes or neurotransmitters, they are present in quantities of a few million molecules, whereas, just one swallow of water containing ONE PART per million of a chemical will contain six hundred quadrillion (600,000,000,000,000) toxic molecules. According to the United States Department of Health, the Tampa Bay area in Florida is the 5th worst area in the nation for polluted water. Also, it should be pointed out that the government, either on the federal, state or local level, cannot possibly supply us with water pure enough for drinking. The cost would be totally prohibitive! You see, only a tiny percentage of water consumption is used for drinking and cooking; most is used for flushing the toilet, watering the lawn, washing dishes, etc. It would be foolish to spend the money to purify water and then flush it down the toilet!

DOMESTIC WATER USES

80 Gallons Per Capita Per Day

Total Indoor Water Use

The time has come when Americans all over this country should exercise their God given authority and provide their families with pure healthful drinking water. The consequences of not doing so will be very expensive in both money and health. What kind of water is best for human consumption and why?

The answer to the first part of that question is short and easy—PURE WATER, H_2O and nothing else. Many books have been written to answer the second part. This question always comes up. Aren't minerals in the water good for me? The answer is an immediate and resounding NO! Your body is designed to assimilate and utilize organic minerals (minerals that come through the food chain). Inorganic minerals can plug up our system. They provide little nutrition. You can't go out in the back yard with a spoon, eat the dirt and expect to get nutrients. The minerals in water are no different. All bottled water labeled Drinking Water, Mineral Water, Spring Water, Natural Water, etc., fall in this category.

Most health experts agree: Drinking impure water contributes to many ailments from simply feeling tired to cancer and heart disease, with many in between like hardening of the arteries, kidney and gall stones, arthritis, gout, high blood pressure and premature aging, while just the opposite is true about PURE water.

BENEFITS OF PURE WATER

1. Pure water can be used by your body directly rather than having to be cleaned and detoxified first, saving a large amount of energy.
2. Pure water cleans toxins and inorganic minerals from your body rather than depositing them in it.
3. All organs, glands and systems in your body function better with plenty of Pure water.
4. The waste disposal organs of your body (colon, kidney, lungs, skin) operate properly only with lots of Pure water. Pure water promotes health—so many of America's most popular beverages rob you of health.

WHAT KIND OF WATER SHOULD I DRINK?

DISTILLED WATER. There are other types of water purifiers but what do the real health experts say? Paul Bragg in *The Shocking Truth About Water*, "Outside of the fruit and vegetable juices, I drink no other water except steam produced distilled water. It is the ideal liquid for efficient functioning of the lungs, stomach, liver and other vital organs."

N.W. Walker in *Water Can Undermine Your Health*, "I can state without fear of contradiction that your Endocrine Glands are by far the most important and vital organs in your body. Your glands NEED Distilled Water!"

Dr. Allen E. Banik, in *The Choice Is Clear*, "The Miracle of all water - Distilled Water! It is God's water for the human race."

Esther Dougherty in *You Have a Right to Know*. "While Distilled water is not to be considered a cure-all, it is without a doubt the best water available to man - and the only truly pure water available in our waste-laden society."

Dr. Paul Conn in *Not a Drop to Drink*, "Distilled Water avoids virtually all the problems of tap water, bottled water, filtered water, well water, and even rain water. It is the ONLY pure form of water."

Perhaps the single, most beneficial lifestyle change needed by most people is simply the daily drinking of large amounts of pure, high energy water!

C.W. DeLavy Evans, M.D. in *How to Prolong Life*, "There is no doubt as to the high value of Distilled Water used freely as a retarder of the ossifying conditions which appear to constitute the condition of old age."

Many other experts on water and health could be quoted, but I think you get the idea. The consensus is clear—*Steam Distilled Water* is the choice. It is not only pure water but high energy water! The distillation process not only removes the impurities but fills the water molecule with the maximum amount of energy it can hold. Therefore, distilled water is much more able to carry nutrients into our system, particularly our liver, than any other type of water. And because the liver must put water, like all types of food energy, on the body's frequency, it is much easier to convert high energy water than low energy water. Then the water can be used by every system and function in our body, particularly the waste removal functions. The scientific explanation of all this is quite fascinating, but beyond the scope of our discussion.

Perhaps the single most beneficial lifestyle change needed by most people is simply the daily drinking of large amounts of pure, high energy water! How much you need depends on how big you are and how hard you work. But everyone should drink at least one half their body weight in ounces every day. That is, if you weigh 200 pounds, drink 100 ounces of water a day.

You owe it to yourself and your family to investigate how the water situation affects you. And do yourself a big favor—drink less coffee, sodas, beer, tap water, etc. and drink much more PURE STEAM DISTILLED WATER.

Most beverages such as colas and coffee don't count toward your daily water consumption because they are full of things that your body has to detoxify and flush out. Coffee, for example, is a diuretic, causing your body to lose more water than you gain. In contrast, whole food concentrate beverages are much different. They contain only nutrients which your body recognizes and quickly utilizes, leaving the pure water to enhance every system and function. Chapter 20 explains this in some detail.

SUMMARY

1. Our water problem is mainly one of quality, not quantity. Although, in recent years it appears that both floods and drought are becoming worse.
2. We should not drink tap water—period!
3. Water is imperative to every function of our body.
4. Steamed distilled water is the best water to drink and cook with.
5. Steamed distilled water is both pure and high energy water.
6. High energy water is the easiest for our body to bring up to its frequency.

THE MOST IMPORTANT SINGLE CHANGE MOST PEOPLE CAN MAKE IS SIMPLY DRINKING ENOUGH PURE, HIGH ENERGY WATER! ! !

16

UNDERSTANDING VITAMINS

I CORINTHIANS 1:25

For the foolishness of God is wiser than man's wisdom, and the weakness of God is stronger than man's strength.

In the nutrition field there is more confusion about vitamins than any other single area. The controversy over vitamins is tremendous. There is so much mis-information and even dis-information that most people simply don't know who to believe.

Over the years I've helped a lot of people improve their health through better lifestyle habits, through better table food selection, through the avoidance of many toxins and poisons and through supplementation with whole food concentrates. By far, the most frequent comment and question I get from new converts goes something like this, "I'm feeling a lot better, but shouldn't I be taking some vitamins?" Over the years we have all been conditioned to think we need massive amounts of vitamins. These synthetic, chemical isolets, unfortunately, have limited vitamin activity in our body, but often turn destructive when taken in excess or in improper ratios (see Chapter 1).

Let's back up a moment. Where do vitamins come from anyway? For thousands of years the only source of vitamins (or any other nutrient) was FOOD—fruits, vegetables, grains, seeds and nuts, as well as meat, eggs and dairy. But, in the last 40 years or so we have found a cheaper source—the pharmaceutical LABORATORY. The vitamins in botanicals, however, remain far superior to synthetic, chemical isolets. I'll use one example; white flour. A wonderful food, like wheat, is stripped of its germ and hull, thereby, removing virtually all of its vitamins, nutrients and fiber. It is processed, refined and bleached. Then a dozen or so artificial vitamins are added back to it and it is then called "enriched". It should be labeled "nutrition free"!

There is one other major source of vitamins—your own body. Friendly bacteria in the colon make vitamins B3, 4, 12 and vitamin K. Sunlight hitting your skin converts cholesterol into vitamin D. Your liver produces Vitamin A from beta carotene. A well-functioning body is a great source of vitamins.

Many vitamins are used as Coenzymes, but for a vitamin to be used as a Coenzyme it must be shaped properly.

Let's review—where do vitamins come from?

1. FOOD
2. YOUR OWN BODY
3. PHARMACEUTICAL LABORATORIES

The first two are very good while the third is very questionable. That brings us to our next question,

How Do Vitamins Work in our Body? Vitamins do thousands of different things in our body. They can be put in three general categories of activities:

1. Coenzymes
2. Carriers, Navigators, Drivers
3. Protectors, Antioxidants

COENZYME ACTIVITY

Many vitamins are used as Coenzymes, but for a vitamin to be used as a Coenzyme it must be shaped properly.

Keeping it extremely simple let's try to understand the concept of coenzyme activity. Every cell in your body is designed to do a very specific job. Many cells perform their function by manufacturing something. It could be insulin, angiotensin, adrenalin, testosterone, serotonin or any other of the thousands of chemicals our bodies make. Each cell knows what it is designed to make because it is under the influence or authority of a particular gene that is part of the DNA that is in the nucleus of every cell. This gene controls an enzyme that is needed to manufacture the chemical produced by that cell. Many times a coenzyme is needed for the manufacturing process. Many vitamins are used as Coenzymes, but for a vitamin to be used as a coenzyme it must be shaped properly!

Many nutrients, including vitamins, work as transport agents to get things where they need to go.

Let's use vitamin C as an example. The chemical name for vitamin C is ascorbic acid. Now, ascorbic acid has four isomers. That is, four molecules with identical parts linked to one another in the same order but arrayed differently in three-dimensional space. The coenzyme action of vitamin C depends upon the shape of its molecule, which fits into a complimentary cavity in the enzymes with which it works, thereby forming a reactive complex. If the ascorbic acid is shaped wrong it will have no vitamin C activity—no coenzyme activity. All plants as they grow make "real" vitamin C—that is, ascorbic acid that is shaped so that it will fit into the body's enzymes.

Well, how important can real vitamins be? Let me use two examples:

1. A substance called carnitine helps to supply the fuel that energizes the contraction of muscle fiber. Its synthesis from the amino acid lysine takes place through five successive reactions, each catalyzed by a specific enzyme. The second and fifth involve hydroxylation, for which vitamin C is needed.
2. In the adrenal glands, enzyme actions mediated by vitamin C, present in large amounts, conver the amino acid tyrosine first to dopa, then to dopamine and then to noradrenaline in the manufacture of the all-important hormone adrenaline.

Have you ever felt very tired for no apparent reason? It may have something to do with the above two examples!, or it may be caused by one of a thousand different activities affecting energy levels. But, it is most likely caused by a combination of several or many imbalances.

CARRIERS, NAVIGATORS, DRIVERS

Many nutrients including vitamins work as transport agents to get things where they need to go. For example, vitamin D carries calcium from the digestive tract into the blood stream. CoQ10 transports oxygen from the cell wall to the mitacondria.

During the last few years there have been more antioxidant supplements put on the market than any other type.

There are many more vitamins that perform these functions than we realize! We all know that beta carotene is important because the liver makes vitamin A out of it. But did you know that beta carotene is just ONE of about 3,000 known carotenoids, all of which are nutrients? The same is true of the tocopherals—vitamin E. There are over 600 bioflavenoids. Do you see the point? When you buy a multiple vitamin supplement, you will be getting massive amounts of synthetic, isolated chemicals that may or may not be shaped right. You will be getting 20 to 30 chemicals. How many vitamins does your body need? Thousands and thousands. In contrast, adequate whole food concentrates provide them all! And since they come from a plant, every one is shaped just right!

PROTECTORS, ANTIOXIDANTS

During the last few years there have been more antioxidant supplements put on the market than any other type. Each new supplement claims almost miracle-like powers by helping the body in so many ways. There are several good reasons for all the recent hype.

First of all, antioxidants are everywhere. There are lots of great botanical sources of antioxidants. In fact, nearly all plants are good sources of antioxidants. So, all an entrepreneur needs to do is find a cheap source of antioxidants, such as grape seeds, write up the horrors of free radical damage, tell how antioxidants help, and he has a strong marketing plan.

Most free radicals should be prevented rather than neutralized. Free radicals come from our polluted air and water, from chemical additives in and on our food and from faulty and incomplete digestion (review Chapter 1). *Drink steamed distilled water...Eat real food...Restore your digestive system...Make sure you have the correct intestinal flora...Eat whole food concentrates!* IF YOU DO THESE THINGS YOU WILL NOT HAVE A FREE RADICAL PROBLEM.

WHY DO WE EAT?

I believe that the correct answer and the original plan was to feed our bodies to maintain a high level of health. Unfortunately, in today's world other answers may apply to many of us:

1. We eat because we are hungry, and we are always hungry because the food we choose is low in nutrients, therefore, not satisfying.
2. We eat for taste, not for nutrition.
3. We eat because we are sad, nervous, anxious or depressed or to 'stuff' some other feeling.
4. We eat because it is time to eat.
5. We eat because it is an appropriate activity at a social occasion.
6. We eat so as not to hurt someone's feelings.

WHY DO YOU EAT?

I have never heard of anyone eating whole food concentrates except to regain or maintain health.

Have you ever gone shopping in a grocery store? Have you ever visited a doctor's office? What was your motivation for going there? Was your motivation the same or different? Most people go to the grocery store to buy food and other products for their daily consumption. Doctor visits are primarily prompted by a crisis situation—when you're sick. Whole food concentrates are like a high quality grocery store, NOT a doctor's office! If you are sick go to a doctor. If you want to maintain a higher level of health, eat the best table food you can find, and supplement with whole food concentrates.

Do you know that your body is capable of regeneration? That means your body can rebuild a weak area and make it strong. When do you think that most regeneration takes place—during times of crisis (sickness) or during times of wellness? Overcoming an illness is crisis management. Rebuilding a weakness is preventative maintenance. The body uses nutrients and energy for both processes. However, regeneration occurs mainly during times of relative wellness. Don't forget to feed your body regenerative nutrition when you are not sick, so you can get healthier and stay that way.

WORDS TO KNOW

Coenzymes

Gene

Enzyme

Isomers

Isolets

SUMMARY

1. Vitamins are essential for our good health. They work as manufacturers, transporters and protectors.
2. Vitamins have to be the right shape.
3. We must have thousands of different vitamins, not just a few major ones. In other words, we need all of the real vitamins.
4. Whole food concentrates are an excellent source of real vitamins.

17

WHAT AND HOW MUCH SHOULD I EAT?

JAMES 4:17

Anyone, then, who knows the good he ought to do and doesn't do it, sins.

Let's work on the second question first. The answer of course is, it depends. It depends on four major aspects of your life;

1. How big you are
2. How old you are
3. How active you are
4. What condition you're in

Let's use an obvious example to get started. When you are at rest, you breathe normally, but when you begin to work, you begin to breathe more deeply and more often. Your body at work requires more oxygen than your body at rest. A 100 pound person requires less food than a 200 pound person to maintain good health, unless that 100 pound person is 13 years old and growing like a weed.

CALORIES

Calories are units of measure, like pounds, or yards or gallons. Calories tell us how much energy is in the food we eat. There are three categories of nutrients that contain calories; carbohydrates, protein and fat. Fat is by far the most efficient form of storing energy. Each gram of fat contains 9 calories, while a gram of both carbohydrate and protein contain 4 calories. A gram is a measure of weight. To give you a perspective, a common paper clip weighs about 1 gram.

So, how much energy (calories) does your body need each day? For the average adult on an average day the following formula will be pretty accurate. Take your ideal weight, add a zero, then multiply that number by 1.25. Example—a lady who should weigh 120 pounds. 120, add a zero = 1200 X 1.25 = 1500 calories a day.

The average American gets far too much fat and protein, while not getting enough complex carbohydrates.

The average American gets far too much fat and protein, while not getting enough complex carbohydrates.

But how many of those calories should come from carbohydrates, protein and fat? I believe the optimum ratio would be 70% complex carbohydrates, 15% protein and 15% fat. In our previous example of 1500 calories per day, it would break down to 1050 calories of complex carbohydrates, 225 calories of protein and 225 calories of fat. Because most food labels and books talk in terms of grams, let's take our example one more step; 262.5 grams of complex carbohydrates, 56 grams of protein and 25 grams of fat.

When a person keeps fairly close to this optimum ratio of energy nutrients, all of the other categories of nutrients seem to take care of themselves. Things like vitamins, minerals, enzymes and fiber.

The Federal Government has researched the area of nutrition and food and come up with a food pyramid that you are probably familiar with. Overall it's pretty good—certainly an improvement over previous efforts. This food pyramid emphasizes a variety of foods starting with grains.

Servings Per Day	Type of Foods
6-11	Grains, bread, cereal, pasta
3-5	Vegetables
2-4	Fruits
2-3	Milk, yogurt, cheese
2-3	Meat, poultry, fish, eggs, nuts
Use Sparingly	Fats, oils, sweets

What Constitutes a Serving?

1 Slice of Bread

1/2 Cup of Rice or Oatmeal

1 Cup of leafy vegetables

1/2 Cup of other vegetables

1 Med. Whole fruit

1/2 Cup canned fruit

1 Cup of milk

1 1/2 oz. of cheese

3 Oz. Meat, poultry or fish

1 Egg

1/2 Cup of beans

3 Oz. of nuts

Fiber is great for weight management because it slows down and limits the absorption of both fats and sugars in the digestive system.

FIBER

Dietary fiber, which not surprisingly, comes mainly in foods high in complex carbohydrate, is an extremely important part of your diet. Here again variety is important because there are a lot of different kinds of fiber. Your body, of course, needs them in the proper ratios and in conjunction with other nutrients. Sharon Fleming, Ph.D., of the University of California at Berkeley says, "Fiber pills are a disaster. They're expensive and to a large degree, ineffective." Apparently isolated fiber supplements don't work like fiber in food. "The physical properties have been altered tremendously, and this can reduce the effectiveness of the fiber, gram for gram," Dr. Fleming explains.

Fiber can be separated into two main categories; soluble and insoluble. Soluble fiber is found in grains, vegetables and fruits and include gums, pectin and hemicellulose. Insoluble fiber is cellulose, lignin, mucilages and hemicellulose in beans, grains, fruits and seeds.

Americans buy nearly 200 million dollars worth of laxatives a year.

An adequate volume and variety of fiber contributes to good health in a great number of ways—everything from protection against constipation to protection against cancer. A huge number of studies proclaim that dietary fiber will help, either directly or indirectly, the great majority of diseases common in our society. Things like heart disease, by lowering LDL cholesterol, all kinds of intestinal disorders such as diverticulosis, and irritable bowel syndrome, Crohn's disease, even ulcers, diabetes, gallstones and many others.

Fiber is also great for weight management because it slows down and limits the absorption of both fats and sugars in the digestive system.

Pectin– slows down the absorption of many foods. It is very good for diabetics. Pectin helps remove many toxins including metals and reduces the risk of gallstones. It is found in many fruits and vegetables like apples, citrus, bananas, carrots, beets, cabbage, peas and okra.

Cellulose– is a carbohydrate that can't be digested by humans. It is good for the removal of trash from the colon—particularly harmful substances from the colon wall. It is found, mostly, in the skins of fruits and vegetables like apples, pears, lima beans, whole grains, carrots, beets, broccoli and Brazil nuts.

Hemicellulose– is an ingestible complex carbohydrate. Because it absorbs water it is like a sponge removing harmful toxins from the digestive tract. Again, it is found in fruits and vegetables like peas, bananas, apples, greens, peppers, beans, corn, cabbage, beets, whole grains and whole grain breads and cereals.

Lignin– will help prevent gallstone formation by binding with bile salts and also lowers cholesterol. It is found in potatoes, tomatoes, green beans, carrots, peas, whole grains, some nuts, peaches, strawberries and other fruits and vegetables.

Mucilages and gums– also help to get rid of toxins and help regulate blood sugar levels. They are found in oatmeal, oat bran, most beans and many seeds.

Did you know that about 20% of the American populace is chronically constipated and that includes the children. Americans buy nearly 200 million dollars worth of laxatives a year. One hundred years ago heart disease was unknown. Cancer and diabetes were extremely rare. Many things have changed—not all for the better; farming methods, food processing, dietary habits and fiber consumption to name a few.

How much fiber is enough? That depends on who you read and who you believe. Some experts recommend up to 50 grams a day. However, nobody is saying less than 25 grams a day. Unfortunately, the average American eats only about 10 grams a day.

Fiber Content of Common Foods

Food	Serving	Fiber in Grams
Beans:		
Black-eyed Peas	1/2 Cup	8.3
Kidney	1/2 Cup	7.9
Chick-Peas	1/2 Cup	7.0
White Beans	1/2 Cup	6.8
Lentils	1/2 Cup	5.2
Pinto Beans	1/2 Cup	4.1
Grains:		
Whole Wheat Bread	1 Slice	2.1
Rye Bread	1 Slice	1.6
White Bread	1 Slice	.5
English Muffin	1	1.6
Bran Muffin	1	3.5
Bagel	1	1.2
Waffle	1	.8
Bran Cereal	2/3 Cup	9.0
Shredded Wheat	2/3 Cup	2.6
Oatmeal	2/3 Cup	1.1
Cornflakes	2/3 Cup	.3

Food	Serving	Fiber in Grams
Fruits:		
Pear	1 Medium	4.2
Strawberries	1 Cup	3.9
Dates	5 Medium	3.5
Orange	1 Medium	3.1
Apple	1 Medium	3.0
Peach	1 Medium	2.3
Banana	1	1.8
Grapes	1 Cup	1.1
Vegetables:		
Peas	1/2 Cup	5.0
Brussels Sprouts	1/2 Cup	3.4
Broccoli	1/2 Cup	3.0
Carrots	1/2 Cup	1.8
Lettuce	1 Cup	1.7
Corn	1/2 Cup	1.2
Cauliflower	1/2 Cup	1.1
Other:		
Most nuts	1/2 Cup	2.5
Meat, poultry, fish		0
Milk, cheese		0
Fats, oils, sweets		0

Fast Food

Is it healthy to eat in fast food restaurants? The answer is generally, NO! That is not to say that the fast food chains are not good corporate members of society—they are. If nobody bought this kind of food, they would not be in business. You don't have to eat there. But from a nutritional point of view they are pretty bad. Extremely high in fat, salt, calories and cholesterol, and extremely low in fiber and balanced nutrition.

Consider these facts on some of the most popular meals in America:

Restaurant	Food Item	Fat (Grms)	Fat %	Calories	Salt (Mg)	Cholesterol (Mg)
McDonald's	Quarter Pounder/cheese	30	51	530	1160	95
McDonald's	Large Fries	22	44	450	290	0
McDonald's	Big Mac	28	47	530	960	80
Burger King	Double Bacon Cheese Burger	39	55	640	1220	145
Burger King	Whopper with Cheese	46	57	730	1300	115
Burger King	Vanilla Shake	7	20	310	230	20
KFC	Extra Crispy Breast	28	54	470	930	80
KFC	Rotisserie Thigh Leg	24	64	333	980	163
Pizza Hut	Personal Pan Pizza Supreme	34	42	722	1760	66
Domino's	2 Slices/Pepperoni Deep Dish	29	42	622	1383	44
Wendy's	Baked Potato /Bacon /Cheese	18	30	540	1430	20
Wendy's	Chicken Sandwich	18	37	440	840	60
Hardee's	Roast Beef	26	56	420	920	50
Hardee's	Omelet Biscuit	30	51	530	1330	175
Taco Bell	Burrito Supreme	19	39	440	1181	45
Taco Bell	Taco Salad	55	58	860	910	80

Let's try to put these fast food meals in perspective. We will use two examples—a 120 pound woman and a 180 pound man.

Optimum DAILY Amounts

	Calories	Fat	Salt	Cholesterol
120 lb. Woman	1500	25 grm.	2400 mg.	300 mg.
180 lb. Man	2250	37.5 grm.	2400 mg.	300 mg.

Eating in fast food restaurants is simply not a healthy thing to do.

If that man ate lunch at McDonald's and had a Quarter Pounder with cheese, large fries and vanilla shake, he would be getting 1290 calories, 59 grams of fat, 1680 milligrams of salt and 115 milligrams of cholesterol in just those three items. That means he would be getting 57.3% of his optimum calories, 157.3% of recommended fat, 70% of his daily sodium allotment and 38.3% of cholesterol.

If our 120 lb. Lady went to KFC and had one extra crispy breast, 1 biscuit, coleslaw and a coke, she would be getting 924 calories, 46 gr. Fat, 1721 mg. salt, 83 mg. cholesterol. Percentage wise her lunch would contain 61.6% of optimum calories, 184% of optimum fat, 71.7% of optimum salt and 27.7% of optimum cholesterol.

Obviously, these meals are much too high in fat and salt, but that is only half the problem. The enormous number of calories provide very little vitamins, minerals, enzymes and complex carbohydrates. Therefore, even though there were too many calories, there were far to few nutrients. This is a classic example of malnutrition, way too much of some things and not nearly enough of others. Meals such as these contribute to free radical formation and damage while providing very little antioxidant protection.

Also, the fat in these meals is easily stored on our bodies, increasing our size and distorting our shape. At the same time that we are gaining weight, we are still hungry, or at least not satisfied, because we are not receiving the great number of nutrients our bodies are calling for.

Eating in fast food restaurants is simply not a healthy thing to do. Did you know that on the average, Americans eat 1/3 of their meals in fast food restaurants? As always, the choice is yours. Of course, these restaurants are exceedingly abundant, conveniently located and open at all hours.

Food Planning

One of the most important habits to develop if you want to be healthy is food planning and preparation. When you get hungry, you are going to eat something. You will either eat what you have planned and prepared or you will eat what is easy and convenient. Easy and convenient almost always means fast foods or unhealthy snacks.

One of the most important habits to develop if you want to be healthy, is food planning and preparation.

The American lifestyle is no longer one of family meals lovingly prepared in the home. The tradition of family communication and sharing around the supper table has been replaced by a trip to McDonald's or order in pizza eaten in front of the T.V. Our nutrition is suffering and so are our family values.

With the great majority of women working outside the home, meal planning and preparation time is at a premium. Therefore, choices must be made. Is it worth the time and effort to eat better? Maybe more people would answer that question in the affirmative if they had better information—if they really knew the significance of their choices. I sincerely hope that is the case and I hope these pages supply some of that information.

Science Magazine recently ran an article about our body rebuilding and replacing itself. According to these researchers, 98% of the atoms in your body are replaced every year. This current research is confirmation of earlier studies that said somewhat the same thing. That is such wonderful news. No matter what we have done in the past, we can be almost 'new' a year from now if we make the right choices day by day.

Phytonutrients

For a long time now, researchers have known that human diets high in grains, beans, vegetables and fruits reduce the risk of getting many diseases like cancer, heart disease, diabetes, hypertension, etc., when compared to diets high in fats, meats and sweets. It is now well recognized that one of the disease-preventing qualities of these natural foods is antioxidants. Antioxidants protect our cells from damage caused by free-radical oxidation. More recently researchers have discovered that these same fruits, vegetables, grains and beans contain another whole group of nutrients that promote health while fighting disease. They are being called Phyto- nutrients.

Phytonutrients, sometimes called phytochemicals are biologically active substances found in plants. Researchers have identified several thousand phytonutrients and new ones are being discovered all the time. No one knows how many phytonutrients there are, but it is estimated that tomatoes alone contain 10,000 different phytonutrients.

New studies concerning phytonutrients are being published every day. Many of these studies are using phytonutrients to fight cancer. There are many examples;

1. Sulforaphane, a phytonutrient found in broccoli, seems to activate enzymes within our cells that will get rid of a potentially carcinogen toxin before it can cause any damage to the cell.
2. Certain Flavonoids found in some fruits and berries, apparently keep some cancer-causing hormones from attacking our cells.
3. Genistein, found in soybeans, prevents capillaries from developing and nourishing tumors, thereby killing the tumor.

4. Indoles, found in cabbage, cauliflower and Brussels sprouts, activate the immune system to excrete from the body, certain carcinogen chemicals.
5. Saponins, found in beans and lentils, seem to prevent cancer cells from multiplying.
6. P-coumaric acid and chlorogenic acid, found in tomatoes block some chemical reactions that would create carcinogens.
7. Phenethyl isothiocyanate, found in turnips and cabbage, apparently protects the lung cell's DNA from carcinogens in tobacco smoke.

These are just seven examples of phytonutrients that scientists now recognize as cancer fighting elements in our natural foods. Do you think science will ever isolate and identify every phytonutrient, and find out how it fights disease and promotes health? If a single vegetable has 10,000 phytonutrients how many are there all together? And that's just considering them individually. We know for sure that nutrients work together. How many possible combinations are there? Fortunately, we don't have to figure it all out! All we have to do is eat a variety of fruits, grains, vegetables and beans. God has already figured it out!

No one knows how many phytonutrients there are, but it is estimated that tomatoes alone contain 10,000 different phytonutrients.

NUTRITION QUIZ

Malnutrition is extremely common in America even among the affluent. Many people would be surprised to learn that they are malnourished. Take this little quiz to see if you are at risk of not getting everything your body needs to be healthy. Be truthful and compare your total score with the format at the bottom of the page.

		Score
1.	I smoke 1/2 pack of cigarettes or more per day.	3
2.	I have more than two drinks of beer, wine or liquor almost every day.	2
3.	I eat in a "fast food" restaurant more than twice a week.	2
4.	I can't always shop, cook or feed myself.	2
5.	I eat less than three meals per day	2
6.	I eat less than two fruits per day.	1
7.	I eat less than four vegetables per day	1
8.	I cook for myself and eat alone most of the time.	1
9.	I don't always have enough money to buy food.	4
10.	I have tooth problems or don't chew my food well.	2
11.	I am more than 25 pounds over weight.	2
12.	I take three or more prescription or over-the-counter drugs per day.	2
13.	I've been in the hospital during the past year.	1

0-2	Keep up the good work. You should be pretty healthy.
3-5	Your risk of malnutrition is moderate. Try to improve right away. The longer you remain at this level the worse the malnutrition will become as your body uses up stored nutrients.
6 or more	Your risk of malnutrition is high. Immediate and substantial steps need to be taken. Remaining at this level will most assuredly lead to illness and disease.

WORDS TO KNOW

Calories

Carbohydrate

Gram

Fiber

Cellulose

Soluble

Insoluble

Phytonutrients

SUMMARY

1. The amount of nutrition you need depends on how big you are, how old you are, how active you are and what condition you're in.
2. Calories are units of measure that tell us how much energy is in the food we eat.
3. Energy containing foods are carbohydrates, proteins and fats.
4. Dietary fiber is extremely important to our health.
5. There are several kinds of necessary fiber that come mostly from whole grains, beans, fruits and vegetables.
6. Fast food is very high in calories, fat and salt and a very poor nutrition source.
7. Phytonutrients are chemical substances in whole foods that our body uses for good health.
8. No one knows how many phytonutrients there are, but several thousand have been identified so far.
9. Take the nutrition quiz to see if you are at risk of malnutrition.

18

TO EAT...OR, NOT TO EAT ?

What to eat is a question each one of us must face three, four, five, six or even more times every day. The choices we make are going to profoundly affect our thinking ability, our attitude, our disposition, our outlook, the way we look, our health and everything else about us.

1 CORINTHIANS 10:31

"So whether you eat or drink or whatever you do, do it all for the glory of God."

A typical American's day might go something like this—get up in the morning and have a cup of coffee or two, skip breakfast; 10:00 A.M., have two donuts and another cup of coffee; for lunch, a super burger, large fries, cola and a piece of pie or cake; about 3:00 P.M., a candy bar and soda; after work, a drink or beer or two; for supper, pork chops, mashed potatoes, canned corn and white bread; while watching TV, cheese and crackers or chips with soda or beer; and ice cream before bed. How is that person's thinking, attitude, disposition, outlook, looks and health going to be?

When you are making your choice, ask yourself these questions, Is this food raw or refined? Was this food made by nature or by man? What is the nutrient to calorie ratio? What is the fat to fiber ratio? Nearly all raw, natural food is very high in nutrients and low in calories while almost all refined and processed foods are high in calories and low in nutrients. We cover many specific foods in other chapters—things like pork, shellfish, salt, blood, animal fat, etc. And we provide you with lists like Clean and Unclean Meat, Snacks,

Dietary No-No's and Ten Best and Ten Worst Foods. We won't try to duplicate those efforts, so this chapter will concern itself with four things; the most outstanding table foods, polyunsaturated fats, colon foods, and a miscellaneous category.

VITAMIN A

Let's talk first about vitamin A. Vitamin A is extremely important in our society for three main reasons:

1. It is necessary for all healing and regeneration to take place.
2. It is necessary to build and maintain healthy skin and mucous membranes, which provides our primary barrier against infections.
3. It is necessary for good vision.

There are two dietary forms of Vitamin A. One is preformed Vitamin A or retinal. Retinal is only found in animal sources and mostly in the fat tissue and liver. The other form is provitamin A or beta-carotene. The original source of retinal is the plant pigment beta-carotene. Beta-carotene supplies more than two-thirds of the Vitamin A in human nutrition.

The liver is by far the most efficient storage organ for Vitamin A, and contains about 90% of the body's total. In a healthy person this is sufficient to supply the body's needs for 6 to 12 months. However, infectious disease and the overuse of antibiotics have severely depleted many people's reserve.

The liver is by far the most efficient storage organ for Vitamin A, and contains about 90% of the body's total.

The following chart shows the ten best food sources for Beta-carotene and the amount of International Units found in $3^{1}/_{2}$ ounces of each food:

Carrots	11,500
Sweet Potatoes	8,800
Spinach	8,100
Cantaloupe	3,400
Apricots	2,700
Broccoli	2,500
Peaches	1,330
Cherries	1,000
Tomatoes	900
Asparagus	900

VITAMIN C

Vitamin C (ascorbic acid) is another very crucial nutrient for health and well-being. The name ascorbic acid was given to this substance because of its anti-ascorbic or anti-scurvy properties. In the normal, healthy individual tissue levels of vitamin C diminish slowly so, with no intake, deficiency symptoms do not appear for approximately three months. Of course, by the time symptoms appear the situation is very serious. Vitamin C is required to build and maintain body tissue in general, including bone matrix, cartilage, dentin, collagen, and connective tissue. Blood vessels particularly are weakened without the cementing effect of vitamin C to provide firm capillary walls. Early deficiency signs include easy bruising, hemorrhages of any kind, poor wound healing and bleeding gums.

Vitamin C is easily destroyed by heat, light and oxidation so the handling, preparation, cooking and processing of any food source of the vitamin should be considered in evaluating that food's contribution of the vitamin to the diet. The following chart shows the ten

Vitamin C is required to build and maintain body tissue. Vitamin C is easily destroyed by heat, light and oxidation.

best food sources of vitamin C and the amount in milligrams found in 3½ ounces of each food:

Bell Peppers	128
Broccoli	113
Brussels sprouts	102
Cauliflower	78
Strawberries	59
Spinach	51
Oranges	50
Cabbage	47
Grapefruit	38
Cantaloupe	33

CALCIUM

There are several "major" minerals needed by the body including; calcium, magnesium, sodium, potassium, phosphorus, sulfur and chlorine. Although they are all important, calcium is probably considered by the general public as the most important; it is certainly the most abundant, with an average 150 pound adult having about three pounds of calcium in their body. Dynamic calcium and phosphorus provide structure for the framework of the body. Free particles of calcium, electrically charged, move about and diffuse through membranes to control a number of body functions like blood clotting, transmission of nerve impulses, muscle contractions and relaxation, membrane permeability and activation of enzymes.

Only about 10% of the calcium in an average diet is absorbed, and sometimes far less. Calcium is insoluble in an alkaline medium so most absorption takes place in the duodenum where the pH is lower. Vitamin D hormone, along with parathyroid hormone are essential for calcium absorption. Excess dietary fat inhibits calcium absorption by forming insoluble calcium soaps, which are excreted along with the calcium. Also, excess fiber in the diet binds calcium. But don't worry about this one because no Americans are likely to fall in this category. In the elderly, in general, and in post-menopausal women in particular, there is a reduced ability to absorb calcium.

The majority of calcium is found in our bones. Bone tissue is constantly being reshaped according to various body needs and stresses, with as much as 700 milligrams of calcium entering and leaving the bones each day.

Excess dietary fat inhibits calcium absorption by forming insoluble calcium soaps, which are excreted.

The following chart shows the ten best food sources of calcium as well as the amount in milligrams in $3^1/_2$ ounces of each food:

Broccoli	103
Spinach	93
Snap Beans	56
Lima Beans	52
Artichokes	51
Cabbage	49
Tangerines	40
Celery	39
Carrots	37
Brussels sprouts	36

I know you were expecting dairy products to be included in the above list. Read Chapter 11 to see why they are not.

ALL NUTRIENTS

We can't take the space here to talk about every vitamin and mineral, obviously they are all vital to good health. Remember, food remains the best source of nutrients. By itself a vitamin can do very little. Its action is catalytic and so it requires a substrate to work on. These necessary substances are the energy nutrients - carbohydrate, fat and protein. The B vitamins, for example, act as vital control agents. They serve in many reactions as coenzyme partners with key cell enzymes in energy metabolism and tissue building.

It is interesting to note that the most nutritious foods were added to mankind's diet after the fall in Genesis, Chapter 3, "The herbs of the field."

Thiamine is needed to produce energy from glucose or to convert it to fat for tissue storage. So too much sugar blows away thiamine. Riboflavin acts as a control agent in both energy production and tissue building. Niacin is a partner with riboflavin in the cellular coenzyme system that converts protein to glucose and oxidizes glucose to release controlled energy. We could go on and on ... but what are the best foods for all of the above? The following chart shows the overall ranking (the ten best foods) based on levels of vitamin A, vitamin C, niacin, riboflavin, thiamine, potassium, iron, calcium, and phosphorus:

Broccoli	Asparagus
Spinach	Artichokes
Brussels sprouts	Cauliflower
Lima beans	Sweet potatoes
Peas	Carrots

Of course, we have been considering familiar, common, available foods. There are many unfamiliar vegetables and herbs that are higher in many nutrients, but you can't go down to your local grocery store and buy them.

The rule of thumb is, the deeper the color in a fruit or vegetable the more nutrition it contains. There are a few exceptions, such as cauliflower in the preceding list. It's interesting to note that the great majority of these foods were added to mankind's diet after the fall in Genesis, Chapter 3, "the herbs of the field."

TASTE

While we are primarily focusing on the nutritional value of food, there is another area of concern for most of us—taste. Most people's taste buds are "turned on" by fat, sugar and salt. It shouldn't come as a big surprise that the tastiest things, when eaten in excess, lead to degenerative disease. The problem is that our taste buds have been overwhelmed by much too much of these very strong flavors, to the point that we can't appreciate the very good but more subtle taste of natural foods.

However, the people who are able to abstain from these strong flavors for a short while are rewarded by a reactivation of their taste buds and a great appreciation of the taste of foods they once considered bland. Of course, their health would automatically improve at the same time.

The properties of garlic that are so good for our health are destroyed when it is deodorized.

There are a great number of wonderful tasting spices that can be added to our foods with no loss of nutrition or detriment to health. Spices like basil, chili powder, oregano, cinnamon, cloves, paprika, bay leaves, cumin, vanilla, sage, curry, cream of tartar and many others.

There are some foods that not only advance your culinary arts but also enhance your health. Products like celery, onions, garlic and cayenne are very good for you. Be careful, there are forces that would destroy the healthful effects of good foods. Take garlic, for example. The properties of garlic that are so good for our health are destroyed when it is deodorized.

Cook with the whole foods whenever you can, but if you buy them in a spice jar, be sure you get the powder form, not the salt form. For example, when making garlic bread, be sure to use garlic powder, not garlic salt. For those who are really hung-up on salt, try these permissible salt substitutes; Bragg's Aminos, Mrs. Dash, Spike and Vege-Sal, in that order. And remember the first rule of good nutrition, "if it tastes good, spit it out". ***Just kidding!***

The two big problems today (as we alluded to earlier) are soil conditions and freshness. By the time fruits and vegetables reach the supermarket, they have traveled an average of 1900 miles. It takes a week for California broccoli to reach a Midwest market, longer to get to Florida. That head of lettuce was probably loaded and unloaded five times. Depending on the season, a peach is less likely to come from Georgia than from Chile; in which case it spends a week or two at sea, a day in fumigation and a day or two on the dock. For each passing day, knock a few points from the nutrition scorecard. It all comes down to time and temperature. Sometimes the big supermarket is better than the health food store because the display cases are colder and the produce moves faster.

COLON FOODS

Let's talk a little bit about foods that are good for the colon. There are some very good natural bowel lubricants. Listed in order of effectiveness they are; flax seed, okra and barley. Adding these to your weekly diet will help. The very best oil for the colon comes from green ripe olives. This is a very special species of olive that is green with dark spots when it is ripe. This olive is excellent at helping to relieve a congested colon and gall bladder. As always, it is far better to eat the whole olive than to eat the refined oil.

Green leafy salads should be made from a variety of leafy vegetables. When eaten before meals, it creates a gelatin like substance from the cellulose that has a bowel cleansing effect. Beets are a good natural laxative food for most people and should be eaten at least once a week - more often during pregnancy. Sauerkraut is very good for a congested colon, particularly when the pH is too high. Don't use the sugared variety. Radishes, watercress, horseradish, hot peppers and cayenne all stimulate digestive speed. Radishes can be used in abundance by children. Pears, either fresh or canned (rinse off the sugar) have a bowel cleansing effect. They have a magnesia compound in them that inhibits the food from adhering to the wall of the colon. They are also very good for the gall bladder. And finally, the bulk contained in such foods as brown rice, dried beans, fruits, vegetables and bran give the colon its needed fiber.

POLYUNSATURATED FATS

We need to talk next about unsaturated and polyunsaturated fats. These are fats that come from vegetable sources like corn oil, soybean oil, etc. Vegetable oils are very refined foods. There are two methods of oil extraction; the mechanical method and the chemical method. The mechanical method goes something like this: The seeds, grains, or beans are crushed then mixed with water and heated to 230° for 30 minutes. Next 20 tons of pressure per square inch is applied to the seeds. Then lye and bleach are added to the oil which is heated to 380° for 12 hours to boil off the chemicals. Usually an antioxidant is added to the final product. The chemical method is much the same except a chemical solvent is used in place of crushing and pressure. Obviously this refining process destroys nearly all nutrients, but we do have nice clear oil. As you know, in the last 30 years vegetable oil has replaced saturated animal fat in our diets to a large extent. As a matter of fact, the average American eats three to four times as much as he used to.

One of the most important habits to develop if you want to be healthy, is food planning and preparation.

When atoms combine to form molecules, their electrons usually group together in pairs. If one of the electrons is lost the molecule becomes a free radical. In the presence of oxygen, free radicals form spontaneously in the tissues from certain substances, like polyunsaturated fat. Free radicals may form in the oil itself while it is still on the shelf or they may form in the tissues once the oil is eaten.

Free radicals can damage nearly every system in the body. When the fine structures and molecules of the cells are damaged, something called lipofuscin pigments are formed. This is the aging process! As the body ages, tissue function decreases, and tissues are unable to maintain and replace themselves. This can easily be seen in older people, for as their hormones, enzymes and antibodies decrease, they become more susceptible to many afflictions. In clinical studies it was found that of those who exclusively ate polyunsaturates, 78% showed marked signs of premature aging—they looked a lot older also.

Polyunsaturated fat inhibits the immune system.

Polyunsaturated fat inhibits the immune system. In fact, it does this so well that researchers are now using polyunsaturated fat in the diets of kidney transplant patients and those with skin grafts taken from other people, so the patients' bodies won't reject the foreign tissue. Another study concluded, "fat seems to have a specific effect in stimulating cancer formation." Premature aging, immune dysfunction, cancer and other health problems have all been linked to increased polyunsaturated fat consumption and its resultant free radical formation.

There seems to be two main reasons why this takes place. First, vegetable oils are highly refined and this refining process destroys virtually all the nutrients. There are certain nutrients which prevent free radical formation. These are called antioxidants. Some primary antioxidants that are abundant in raw foods but absent in refined oils are Vitamins A, C and E, as well as the mineral selenium. The other problem is the actual shape of the polyunsaturated fat molecule. The natural and proper shape of the fat molecule is a horseshoe; this is called a "cis" fat. During the refining process and particularly when the oil is hydrogenated (to make it solid at room temperature) some of the natural horseshoe shapes are changed to straight shapes called trans fats. Liquid oil has about 6% "trans" fats, margarine 54% trans fats and shortening 58% trans fats.

When our cells try to build a good wall around themselves and have to use straight shapes when the blueprint calls for horseshoe shapes, the wall is not going to be very strong. Weak cell membranes make for weak cells—much more susceptible to free radicals and disease.

Finally, a very, very brief discussion on the other two highly refined products we eat so much of and that are, therefore, so detrimental—sugar and white flour.

Sugar is so bad because we eat so much of it! The average American eats over 160 lbs of sugar every year. Sugar is totally devoid of nutrients and is 100% calories. Sugar is a contributing cause of cardiovascular disease, diabetes, cancer, hypertension, tooth decay and obesity. It is a drug and very addictive. It uses up the body's supply of thiamine and chromium and thereby invites disease both physical and mental.

(See chapter 10)

White flour is refined flour and should not be eaten. During the milling process the germ is removed, and the germ contains most of the nutrients. Also, the hull or bran is removed and with it goes the dietary fiber. All that is left is a white powder that when mixed with water makes paste and clogs up our digestive tract. It simply adds unneeded calories and takes away our desire for wholesome nutritious foods.

If you want to be strong and healthy choose foods from nature's banquet table and stay away from artificial, refined, processed and man-made foods.

DIETARY NO-NO'S

Anyone desiring to raise their level of health would do well to review their basic dietary choices. Although the following list is among America's "most popular" foods, they are also among the poorest choices we can make. They lead to degenerative disease rather than abundant health.

1. **White flour:** white bread, rolls, buns, white pasta, etc.
2. **Refined vegetable oil**
3. **Sugar and sugar snacks and desserts:** candy, candy bars, granola bars, doughnuts, rolls, cakes, pies, etc.
4. **Soda pop:** regular or diet, all brands.
5. **Salt and salty snacks:** pretzels, chips, salted nuts, salted popcorn, etc.
6. **All processed and refined foods:** they are loaded with salt, sugar, chemicals, preservatives, dyes, etc., while most nutrients have been removed or destroyed.
7. **"Fast Foods":** If you want to be healthy stay out of fast food restaurants.
8. **Excess protein:** meat, chicken, fish, dairy, eggs, protein powders.
9. **Fat:** red meat fat, chicken skin.
10. **Blood:** meat with the blood in it.
11. **Unclean meat:** pork, shellfish, catfish, etc.
12. **Dark cheeses:** white or very light yellow cheeses are permissible in moderation, less of any of it is best.
13. **Caffeine:** coffee, coke, chocolate, etc.
14. **White potatoes:** as French fries, potato chips, etc.
15. **Most dry, cold breakfast cereals:** contain salt, sugar and fat.
16. **Alcohol:** beer, wine, liquor (except in extreme moderation).
17. **Tobacco:** cigarettes, cigars, pipe, snuff, chewing tobacco.

TEN OF THE BEST FOODS

Broccoli and carrots: High fiber, high vitamins, low calories, possible protection against cancer

Oats: Protein, cholesterol-reducing fiber

Cabbage family: (cabbage, cauliflower, Brussels sprouts, Kale)—Vitamins, reduce risk of colon cancer

Sweet Potatoes: Low calories (unless you add butter or sour cream), high in nutrients

Fresh fruit: Fiber, vitamins, minerals

Dried peas and beans: High fiber, reduces cholesterol; Lentils among the best

Pasta - Artichoke, Whole Wheat, Spinach: Protein, vitamins, minerals—but watch the sauces

Whole-Grain Bread

Scale Fish: Helps prevent heart disease

Yogurt: Friendly bacteria plus pretty good nutrients

...and a bonus: **Popcorn:** (unbuttered)—fiber for only 23 calories a cup

TEN OF THE WORST FOODS

Soda Pop: Sugar or Aspartame, coloring, no nutrition

French Fries: Triple the calories of a baked potato, loaded with oxidized fat

Potato Chips: "You might as well drink a glass of grease." Baked is much better

Bacon: 95% of its calories come from fat. High in salt and cancer-causing nitrates and nitrites

Fettucine Alfredo: Pasta drowned in a sea of fat

"Super burgers": (Big Macs, Whoppers, Checkers, etc.) - Lots of sodium and 600 calories, half from fat

Granola Bars: High fat, high sugar—no better than a candy bar

Sugary Cereals: "Candy with milk on it"

Doughnuts: Again, fat and sugar. Worse than no breakfast at all

Cheese: Fat, cholesterol, salt. But some are better: cottage cheese, part-skim mozzarella, part- skim ricotta, feta, Swiss

SUMMARY

1. When making food choices ask yourself these questions. What is the nutrient to calorie ratio? What is the fat to fiber ratio? Was the food made by nature or by man?
2. Some of the most nutritious common foods are broccoli, spinach, Brussels Sprouts, lima beans, peas, asparagus, artichokes, cauliflower, sweet potatoes, carrots.
3. Fat, sugar and salt taste good, but are destructive when we eat too much. Example: a donut tastes good but is mostly fat and sugar.
4. Polyunsaturated fat is bad for many reasons.
5. The average American eats over 160 pounds of sugar every year.
6. White flour is good for making paste, not for making food.

19

BODY, MIND COUPLING

During my years as a nutritional counselor there has been one nearly universal request, "what can I take to get rid of the fog I'm in?" "Give me a memory pill." "How can I get my ambition back?" "I feel tired and dull all the time." These and other similar questions and comments coming from people of all ages, even in their 20's and 30's, point out the wide spread desire for the return of an alert and active mind for many people.

Chances are very good that you also feel that way some of the time. You might feel groggy when you get up in the morning. Maybe you don't come alive until you've had a couple of cups of coffee. Do you have total instant recall? Most people don't. Have you ever been asked a question and replied, "I know that. Wait. Don't tell me. It's on the tip of my tongue. It starts with a T." Then you remember it during lunch three hours later. Many of us are not as sharp and not as clear as we used to be. We're not as curious or as adventuresome. We feel 'down in the dumps' too much. We're not happy, and we don't get along with people as well. We sometimes feel confused and easily distracted. We have difficulty making up our minds, and when we do we can't stick to it. We might have headaches or equilibrium problems. And, many of us end up worried, moody, anxious or depressed.

2 PETER 3:1

Dear friends, this is now my second letter to you. I have written both of them as reminders to stimulate you to wholesome thinking.

Have you ever stopped to really consider where your brain stops and your mind begins? Your brain is every bit as much of a physical organ as your kidneys or your liver. It is a massive organ made of billions of cells, doing millions of functions for the body, but it transcends the physical and is the seat of the mental processes or reasoning and thinking, of our will, and of our emotions. Christians call this part of us, the soul.

Have you ever stopped to really consider where your brain stops and your mind begins?

I believe that the Bible teaches that we are a trichotomy, that is, we are body, soul and spirit. Some think that the soul and spirit are the same thing, but Hebrews 4:12 says, "for the Word of God…penetrates even to dividing soul and spirit …". When we think of our soul as our thinking capacity, our emotions and our will, the 23rd Psalm takes on added emphasis. "He restoreth my thinking." "He restoreth my emotions." "He restoreth my will." "He restoreth my mental health."

This whole area of man's soul and the power of the soul is exceedingly interesting. Genesis 2:7 says, "and the Lord God formed man of the dust of the ground, and breathed into his nostrils the breath of life; and man became a living soul."

Our spirit is that part of us that makes us conscious of God and relates us to Him. Our body relates us to the world. Our soul relates us to ourselves, or makes us conscious of ourselves. God created Adam, and therefore mankind, with tremendous soul power. That is, he was super intelligent with enormous mental abilities. Adam named every creature on the earth (Genesis 2:19). Adam managed and administered the garden of Eden, an area of hundreds of thousands of square miles (Genesis 2:15).

Then came "the fall." Adam and Eve sinned against God and death entered the world. You know the story of how Satan tempted Eve, but what part of mankind died? Apparently, it was the spirit; that part that gives us God-consciousness. When Jesus was teaching Nicodemus in John, Chapter 3, He said, "I tell you the truth, no one can enter the kingdom of God unless he is born of water and the Spirit. Flesh gives birth to flesh, but the Spirit gives birth to spirit." Paul clarified the matter in 1 Corinthians 15:45, "So it is written: 'The first man, Adam, became a living soul,' the last Adam, a life-giving spirit." The "last Adam," of course, is Jesus Christ.

At "the fall," many things happened; including mankind's losing the use of most of his soul power. Apparently, God somehow hid man's soul power in man's fleshly body. Throughout history there has been evidence of man's hidden soul power coming through. Remember in Exodus, Chapter 7, when the Egyptian magicians turned their staffs into snakes?

Our Spirit is that part of us that makes us conscious of God and relates us to Him.

Today, a great number of people are trying to liberate their hidden soul power. We even have a science dedicated to that purpose. It's called parapsychology. These soul power endeavors would include things like, extrasensory perception, mental telepathy, hypnotism, neurology, psychometry, telekinesis, clairvoyance, astroprojection, and the like. Black magic, witchcraft and voodoo are in the same category but with an obviously wicked connotation.

Many of the world's religions are really based on and seek after this soul power. The abstract meditation of the Taoists, the ascetic practices of the Buddhists, the transcendental meditation of the Hindu are three examples. They all recognize the potential power within mankind and mistakenly believe that god is imprisoned inside us. Some even teach that this inner power will allow us to become gods.

The Bible, however, repeatedly warns us against seeking this soul power. Remember, it brings self-consciousness, not God-consciousness. Can you imagine what would happen if mankind in his present, depraved moral condition, became fully empowered in all his potential psychic abilities? It would be like giving biological, chemical and atomic weapons to psychopaths.

Scripture tells us that God wants to renew our spirit. (Ezekiel 36:26, John 3:6, Ephesians 5:18). Scripture also tells us to rely on God and His power for everything we need. Even Jesus, when on earth, did nothing except what the Father wanted (Matthew 26:39, John 6:38).

Today, a great number of people are trying to liberate their hidden soul power.

Satan, however, wants the use of man's soul power. Isn't that one reason he tempted Eve in the first place? It appears that Satan will indeed control this soul power or at least some of it. The Bible warns us about the use of "great signs" and "lying wonders" (Matthew 24:24, 2 Thessalonians 2:8-10, Revelation 13:25). In Revelation 18:11-13, we are told that souls of men will even be commodities to be traded. Matthew 24:22 says, "If those days had not been cut short, no one would survive, but for the sake of the elect those days will be shortened."

God wants us to be in good mental health, to be in control of our emotions and our thinking and to be active and adventuresome. He does not want us to seek psychic powers or to put our will before His will. If we are to prosper, we really must do things God's way.

BRAIN FUNCTION

A doctor would call lowered brain function "chronic cerebral insufficiency." That just means our brain doesn't work as well as it should. As we get older we expect some of these things to happen, we even consider it normal. But wait a minute! Cancer and heart disease occur more often to older people, and that sure isn't normal. So these things are not necessarily a sign of aging, but a degeneration of the brain. Now, that might seem like pessimistic news, but it's really quite the opposite because degeneration, as opposed to normal aging, can be prevented and reversed.

In your brain are a lot of special cells called neurons. Each neuron has tiny fibers protruding from their wall, with bulbs at their ends. A chemical bursts out of a bulb and attaches to an adjoining cell, charging it with electricity. This chemical is a neurotransmitter. It is the reason you can read and understand these words. The genes inside the cells direct the production of the neurotransmitters. Neurotransmitters control your IQ, that is, your learning, memory and intelligence. But they do much more than that. They enable you to go to sleep or to wake up. They influence your sex drive, your dreams and your appetite. They make you calm or tense, happy or sad. They even control your muscles. In fact, you can't do a thing without them. So, these brain chemicals control our mental and physical processes, but what controls the chemicals? Two basic things, diet and your predominant thinking patterns.

DIET AND THINKING

There are a number of neurotransmitters or brain chemicals that allow our thinking and other brain functions. They have names like serotonin, dopamine and acetylcholine, to name a few. These brain chemicals are extremely diet dependent. For example, choline is one nutrient necessary for our cells to make acetylcholine. Choline is found in lecithin. Some therapists, therefore, use lecithin in treating Alzheimer's disease.

Obviously, malnutrition could affect the production of these essential brain chemicals, but there is another big problem—brain energy! Our brain must generate a lot of energy because it uses a lot of energy. Brain energy production is different from energy production in the rest of our body. Our brain requires at least 40 different nutrients for optimal energy production and a lack of any one of them will disrupt or slow down the production of energy.

When there is a shortage of brain energy, our "thinking" suffers most. Our conscious thinking occurs in the cerebral cortex part of our brain. Other parts of our brain handle the automatic functions for our body through the autonomic nervous system. Thank goodness we don't have to think about liver function or kidney function—that's all automatic. Scientists have determined that the cerebral cortex uses up to twice as much energy as other parts of our brain. That's good for the body, but it can be bad for our learning ability, memory, concentration and our ability to control our emotions.

Our brain requires at least 40 different nutrients for optimal energy production.

Did you know that your emotions are centered in the limbic part of your brain? Did you know that your ability to control your emotions is in the cortex or thinking part of your brain? What happens when there is a shortage of brain energy? Your emotions can be fully energized while your ability to control those emotions can be under-energized. All this from poor nutrition.

Sugar seems to be one of the worst villains in this scenario because so many people eat so much of it. Sugar promotes inappropriate brain chemical production which leads to imbalances. Sugar uses up a lot of nutrients desperately needed for other functions. Sugar laden foods take the place of nutritious foods in many people's diet.

Without ample supplies of certain key nutrients, the neurotransmitters don't get made and when they don't get made, we don't think well. Brain function depends very much on what you ate at your last meal! Recent studies have shown that undernutrition and isolation result in a lack of interest, apathy, and a reduction in outgoing behavior. Add to this the fact that many toxins have an affinity for brain and nerve cells and interrupt normal function when stored there.

THINKING PATTERNS

By thinking patterns, I mean the kind of thoughts you hold in your mind most of the time. Are they worrisome, fearful, pessimistic, negative and anxious? How about angry, bitter, covetous, or unforgiving? The Bible warns us not to think that way. Matthew 6:31-33 says, "So do not worry, saying, 'What shall we eat?' or 'What shall we drink?' or 'What shall we wear?' For the pagans run after all these things, and your heavenly Father knows that you need them. But seek first His kingdom and His righteousness, and all these things will be given to you as well."

Worry is unhealthy. Worry causes imbalances in our brain and in our body. Worry can literally make us sick. We place in our minds whatever we choose to think about—fearful and pessimistic or hopeful and optimistic. The Bible tells us in II Corinthians 10:5, "We demolish arguments and every pretension that sets itself up against the knowledge of God, and we take captive every THOUGHT to make it obedient to Christ."

Whatever we think about, our mind will try to make happen.

We can hold worrisome, fearful and pessimistic thoughts in our mind or we can think about positive, constructive and beneficial things. Whatever we think about, our mind will try to make happen. That's the way it's been designed! Can you now begin to see why goal setting might be important?

One way our body responds to worry is by making extra endorphins. Endorphins are narcotic chemicals, natural pain killers, that when in excess can dull us mentally and emotionally and even bring on depression. Endorphins have a tendency to deactivate the hippocampus. The hippocampus is the brain center for learning and memory. Therefore, endorphins can reduce learning and concentration. They also can make us dull, unable to pay attention.

Some people worry and get depressed, other people worry and become anxious. It doesn't really matter which imbalance is generated because either imbalance affects us the same way. It seems that we need to be calmly aroused for our best learning, memory and alertness. Balance, again, is the key. Worry, fear, negativity and pessimism bring on imbalance, while positive, optimistic thoughts help us maintain balance.

ATTITUDE

by

Charles Swindoll

The longer I live, the more I realize the impact of attitude on life. Attitude, to me is more important than facts. It is more important than the past, than education, than money, than circumstances, than failure, than successes, than what other people think or say or do. It is more important than appearance, giftedness or skill. It will make or break a company…a church…a home. The remarkable thing is we have a choice every day regarding the attitude we will embrace for that day. We cannot change our past…we cannot change the fact that people will act a certain way. We cannot change the inevitable. The only thing we can do is play on the one string we have, and that is our attitude…I am convinced that life is 10% what happens to me and 90% how I react to it. And so it is with you…We are in charge of our Attitudes.

You have probably heard that we have two sides to our brain; the left side and the right side. Our left brain is logical and our right side is intuitive. You might have heard the expression, "He is a right brain thinker" or "She is left brained." The left brain of a mathematician is no doubt more prominent while in an artist the right brain probably would dominate. However, everyone needs to use both sides of their brain, particularly in problem solving. When we learn and remember, we must first sort and categorize things and then give them meaning by comparing them to our past experience. Our left brain categorizes, our right brain gives meaning. Apparently we can't be logical and intuitive at the same time. So, our brain cycles quickly back and forth between right side and left side. This all ties in with the calmly aroused principle, because the right brain is connected to our calming side called the parasympathetic nervous system while the left brain is connected to our arousal side called the sympathetic nervous system. As you can see, we have been designed with two halves to our nature—our sympathetic half and our parasympathetic half. Our sympathetic half does our work; our parasympathetic half restores our capacity to work. This cycling back and forth between working and restoring is needed for success; balance is essential!

This cycling back and forth between working and restoring is needed for success; balance is essential.

When we were born our parasympathetic system came fully developed. That's our restoring half—the one responsible for eating, drinking, sleeping and getting rid of wastes. In contrast, our sympathetic nature must be developed. As infants we were naturally curious so we explored or worked. Unfortunately, our exploring had its risks and as we grew we gradually found our curiosity replaced by fear. Over time we learned to worry and think negative, pessimistic thoughts.

These kinds of thoughts, as we have just learned, bring on the imbalances of depression or anxiety. Anxiety or depression contribute to brain chemicals being either underproduced or produced in excess. Do you see the vicious cycle here? Right thinking and goal setting have the opposite effect—they encourage balance.

Remember the hippocampus? It is partially responsible for controlling the balance between arousal and calmness. This fact takes on special significance when we learn that the hippocampus is the part of the brain that handles novelty. All new experiences (learning) get routed through the hippocampus.

When imbalances get really bad, they can bring on a sense of helplessness. It is essential to understand that this sense of helplessness is a product of our mind, not a product of our circumstances!! Scientists have illustrated this point many times with experimental animals. They have subjected animals to unpleasant situations over which they have no control. Things like forced swims in cold water. At some point the animal will 'give up,' it will have learned helplessness. This is the exact time when certain hormones get out of balance. Some are over produced, some are underproduced. The normal cycles of these hormones are not linked in the proper and normal and healthy way. This hormone shift is a physical footprint of the 'helpless' state. Then when the animal is taken out of that environment and placed back in normal surroundings, it will still exhibit the symptoms of helplessness. The helplessness has gone from the physical realm to the mental realm. Most of us have learned some degree of helplessness as we were growing up! Most helplessness does not come from our circumstances but from our memory. We interpret our present situation in terms of our past experiences and we 'see' only what our memories allow. Therefore, our view of the way things are may be incorrect even though we are convinced they are correct. When this happens, we act or fail to act because of our illusion, not because of the truth.

We interpret our present situation in terms of our past experiences and we *see* only what our memories allow.

Perhaps the hardest concept for understanding our body-mind coupling is the mathematical definition of information. Practically speaking, information and energy are different forms of the same thing, energy being physical, information being mental.

In 1921 Albert Einstein won the Nobel Prize for his complicated mathematics of thermodynamic energy.

During WWII a man named Claude Shannon was using some of Einstein's formulas to solve some military radar problems. Mr. Shannon found that his mathematical expressions of information were the same as Einstein's for energy. F.M. Harold put it this way in his book The Vital Force: A Study of Bioenergetics, "...one may loosely think of information as a special kind of energy required for the work of establishing order. (Remember the Second Law of Thermodynamics).

Information or knowledge or wisdom is the energy we have for use by our minds

The Bible doesn't use the word information. It uses two words that contain the concept of information that we are speaking of here; they are knowledge and wisdom.

Proverbs 3:11-15: "My son, do not despise the Lord's discipline and do not resent His rebuke, because the Lord disciplines those He loves, as a father the son he delights in. Blessed is the man who finds wisdom, the man who gains understanding for she is more profitable than silver and yields better returns than gold. She is more precious than rubies; nothing you desire can compare with her."

So, information or knowledge or wisdom is the energy we have for use by our mind!

The Bible also teaches us that the way to gain information is to be actively involved with our environment, exploring it with all our faculties. (Reread the verses above). Isn't that what James is talking about in James 1:2-4 (Amplified Bible): "Consider it wholly joyful, my brethren, whenever you are enveloped in or encounter trials of any sort or fall into various temptations. Be assured and understand that the trial and proving of your faith bring out endurance and steadfastness and patience. But let endurance and steadfastness and patience have full play and do a thorough work, so that you may be (people) perfectly and fully developed (with no defects), lacking in nothing."

Can you begin to see why God allows us to be in trying circumstances? To gain information (wisdom)

which is mental energy. Does the Bible give us hope and encouragement in those situations? How about Matthew 7:7-8, (Amplified): "Keep on asking and it will be given you; keep on seeking and you will find; keep on knocking (reverently) and the door will be opened to you. For everyone who keeps on asking receives; and he who keeps on seeking finds; and to him who keeps on knocking, the door will be opened."

James 1:5 says, "If any of you is deficient in wisdom, let him ask of the giving God (who gives) to everyone liberally and ungrudgingly, without reproaching or faultfinding, and it will be given him."

Let's say that a man suddenly finds himself in one of those trials James talks about—he discovers he has cancer. I believe his actions, his attitude and his thinking patterns will have a great effect on the situation. If his thoughts are fearful and helpless, if his attitude is complaining and pessimistic, then his chances for recovery are greatly diminished. Even if his attitude is great and his thoughts are positive, it may not be enough if done incorrectly.

Rather than positively and aggressively thinking about getting rid of the cancer, he should positively and aggressively imagine himself in perfect health! Do you see the difference?

So the answer to this active and alert mind dilemma is very simple but certainly not easy: THINK RIGHT AND EAT RIGHT!!!

We need to eat a large variety of fresh, whole foods. Next most important is the whole food and herbal concentrates that are covered extensively in the next chapter. They are without a doubt the best supplements.

While our emotions of helplessness and our memories are real, helplessness itself is not real. Challenges are to be faced and overcome. Consider this, the anecdote for helplessness may be helpfulness.

WORDS TO KNOW

Soul

Autonomic Nervous System

Lecithin

Cerebral Cortex

Neurotransmitter

Sympathetic

Neurons

Limbic System

Parasympathetic

SUMMARY

1. Many people are not mentally sharp and clear.
2. Some brain chemicals are called neurotransmitters.
3. Brain chemicals are very diet-dependent.
4. Brain energy production requires at least 40 nutrients.
5. Our thinking ability controls our emotions.
6. Sugar is bad for our brain.
7. Worry and other bad thoughts are destructive.
8. Our brain and mind must balance in all of their aspects.
9. We need to be calmly aroused.
10. Helplessness is usually mental, not actual.
11. Information is energy for our mind.
12. We need to control our thoughts.
13. Right thinking and right eating bring balance and health.

20

WHY EAT WHOLE FOOD CONCENTRATES?

PROVERBS 13:16

Every prudent man acts out of knowledge, but a fool exposes his folly.

The answer to that question is exceedingly simple—to become and/or remain more healthy!

However, the great majority of Americans have a lot of difficulty understanding and believing why whole food and herbal concentrates promote health. That is because of our heritage. Twentieth Century Americans have been brought up to believe they can eat whatever they want, and when they get sick the doctor will cure them.

Although the evidence has been apparent for decades, it has only been within the last few years that some people have become convinced of our erroneous thinking. The truth is now accepted by many, and the tide of that truth will undoubtedly sweep across America in the 21st Century. The human body is designed to eat food, not chemicals. Health is a body in balance, and balance can only be achieved through proper nutrition, physical exercise and correct thinking.

Did you know that many Americans today are suffering from dangerous nutritional deficiencies which cannot be remedied by simply eating more food because the soil is so depleted? The alarming fact is that nearly all foods are now being raised on land that no longer contains enough needed minerals. Our food is inadequate no matter how much of it we eat! However, at the same time many of those same Americans are suffering certain nutritional overloads caused by inappropriate supplementation. Most processed foods are "enriched" with synthetic chemical isolate vitamins and inorganic minerals. Also, many people are taking mega-doses of synthetic vitamins and hormones with complete disregard of proper balance.

Our forefathers could thrive on a selection of foods that today would cause us to become malnourished.

You'd think, wouldn't you, that a carrot is a carrot, that one is about as good as another as far as nourishment is concerned? But it isn't. One carrot may look like another, yet be lacking in the particular mineral elements which our body requires and which carrots are supposed to contain. Laboratory tests prove that the fruits, the vegetables, the grains, the eggs and the milk and meats of today are not what they were a few generations ago. This undoubtedly explains why our forefathers could thrive on a selection of foods that today, would cause us to become malnourished. The average American of today can not eat enough fruits and vegetables to supply his system with the mineral salts he requires for perfect health because his stomach isn't big enough to hold them. And most of our stomachs are too large already. The truth is that our foods vary enormously in value, and some of them aren't worth eating as food.

The prophet Isaiah warned us that the earth would wear out and he told us why. Isaiah 24:4-5 says, "The earth dries up and withers, the world languishes and withers, the exalted of the earth languish. The earth is defiled by its people; they have disobeyed the laws, violated the statutes and broken the everlasting covenant". And again, Isaiah 51:6 says, "Lift up your eyes to the heavens, look at the earth beneath; the heavens will vanish like smoke, *the earth will wear out like a garment* and its inhabitants die like flies". Hebrews 1:10-11 says, "In the beginning, O Lord, you laid the foundations of the earth, and the heavens are the work of your hands. They will perish, but you remain; they will wear out like a garment."

It shouldn't have to be that way. As a matter of fact, it wasn't supposed to be that way. It has taken man many years of improper farming methods to ruin our soils. But nature can and will solve this problem if she is encouraged to do so. However, until the time comes when man recognizes his folly and starts rebuilding the soil, supplementing our diet with whole food concentrates is the decision of choice for the well informed seeker of health.

Laboratory tests have proved over and over again that our foods simply don't contain the nutrients necessary to keep us healthy.

The need for nutrients of all kinds, particularly minerals, has been demonstrated beyond any doubt over the last 80 years or so. It is now agreed that scores of mineral elements are indispensable for good health. Among the best documented are calcium, potassium, iron, phosphorus, iodine, zinc, etc. A 10-year test with rats proved that by withholding calcium, they can be bred down to a third the size of those fed with an adequate amount of that mineral. Their intelligence, too, can be controlled by mineral feeding as readily as can their size, their bony structure and their general health.

By re-establishing a proper soil balance crops can be grown that contain an ample amount of the desired minerals. It has been proven again and again that crops grown in a properly mineralized soil are bigger and better; that seeds germinate quicker, grow more rapidly and make larger plants; that trees are healthier and bear more fruit of better quality.

Remember the story of the Israelites when they were delivered out of Egypt and went up to the promised land? They sent some men in to spy out the land. In Numbers 13:23 it says, "When they reached the Valley of Eshcol, they cut off a branch bearing a single cluster of grapes. Two of them carried it on a pole between them, along with some pomegranates and figs." The food back then was not only large, but full of all of the great nutrients that God intended.

A healthy plant grown in soil properly balanced can and will resist most insect pests. That very characteristic makes it a better food product. You may have tuberculosis and pneumonia germs in your system, but you're strong enough to throw them off. Similarly, a really healthy plant will pretty nearly take care of itself in the battle against insects and blight—and will also give the human system what it requires. This was shown to be true by Dr. Northern in the 1930's when he grew tomato and cucumber plants, both healthy and diseased, where the vines intertwined. The bugs ate up the weak plants but refused to touch the healthy plants. Such foods keep much better, with and without refrigeration, proving that the cell structure is sounder.

All the nutrients in whole food work together better than each part would separately.

Laboratory tests have proved over and over again that our foods simply don't contain the nutrients necessary to keep us healthy. It shouldn't be that way, but it is. What should we do about it? Grow all our own food in an organic garden? That's one excellent solution, but how many of us are ready for that? No, supplementation is the answer for most of us. So the next question is what kind of supplements? Or does it make any difference? YES ! ! ! Here's why…SYNERGY!

Synergy means that the total is greater than the sum of its parts. If there were synergy in mathematics, which there is not, then 1 + 1 might equal 3. This is a very important concept when it comes to feeding our body. You see, whole foods are synergistic when they are eaten. That is, all the nutrients in the whole food work together better than each part would separately. The nutrients are in the proper form, combination and ratio to build or regenerate the body.

Let's use an analogy to enhance our understanding of synergy. Picture yourself remodeling your living room. You have everything removed right down to the studs, and you are ready to order the drywall. At that point you could call the lumber yard and tell them you have a 12 X 20 foot room that needs drywall, please deliver the proper amount. Pretty soon the truck would come and you would have a pile of drywall in the middle of the room. Is that where you want it? That's like taking an individual vitamin or mineral, it's there in the house, but it's not on the walls. Rather than the lumber yard you could call a drywall contractor who would not only bring the drywall, but all the tools to hang it and the men to do the job. The contractor, of course, is like whole foods or whole food concentrates that have the synergy to do the total job. Of course, if you have the proper tools, experience, and help, you can put up the drywall yourself, but lacking any of those required parts will probably cause a less than perfect job to be done. The same with your body. It can go out and find all the other nutrients to perform that certain function, and assuming there are no nutritional deficiencies, the job might eventually get done. However, that is not the most efficient way. And since our present day foods have been shown to be lacking in nutrients because of poor soil conditions, whole food concentrates are perhaps the best alternative.

There is an amazing array of nutritional supplements on the market. So much so, in fact, that anyone can become confused. Let's try to simplify things. First of all, try not to use anything synthetic! Our body can best use natural, organic nutrients, not synthetic chemicals. If it came out of a lab and not out of a food, it's synthetic. That will eliminate the great majority of products. Next, look for supplements that have nature's synergy built in. These will be whole food concentrates. Nutrients combined by man in the laboratory do not have synergy! That means that multiple vitamins or multiple mineral supplements do not have synergy and should be used only in specific instances of deficiencies or need.

Simply put, whole food concentrates are always 100% natural. They never use synthetic anything! They should come from organically grown fruits, vegetables and herbs. Fruits, vegetables and herbs should never be sprayed with insecticides, herbicides, fungicides, rodentcides, or chemical fertilizers. Produce should be handled very carefully to retain the nutrients as well as the total synergy available in the foods. Because of these facts, and because the whole food concentrates need less digestion, they are available to the body much faster and more completely than other products and even better than the foods they come from. Also, some formulas are system specific. That means they contain the nutrients needed by a particular system of the body, like the immune system or the digestive system, etc.

The scientific method is great for certain things but it's not good for whole foods.

When it comes to nourishing our bodies, a large variety of foods grown in rich organic soil, using no insecticides, herbicides, pesticides, or other chemicals and allowed to ripen on the plant and eaten fresh, is by far the best choice. However, given the present state of our soils and farming methods, the food we have available is inadequate to support optimal health! One excellent answer to this dilemma is whole food concentrates to meet the nutritional needs of your body.

Unfortunately, the world's system has turned to man-made substitutes instead.

How could such a knowledgeable and intelligent society like the United States wander so far away from the principle of regenerating the body's ability to perform its own functions rather than substituting for the body's functions? That mystery isn't hard to solve. It happened little by little over the past 100 years or so, as the scientific method of inquiry has gained strength in the investigations of the natural sciences.

Paradoxically, perhaps it all started with the discovery of vitamins. Early researchers stumbled upon the idea that certain diseases like scurvy and beri-beri might be caused by something being absent in the diet of the victim. For example, when researchers fed chickens refined, white rice, the chickens got sick and died, but when fed whole grain brown rice, they got well and thrived. By further research the scientists were able to ISOLATE a substance we now call Thiamine (vitamin B-1), the absence of which was primarily responsible for the beri-beri-like disease that was affecting the chickens. From that time until this the practice of breaking a substance down to its smallest parts (isolating), then making that part in the laboratory (synthesizing) and very carefully controlling the amount of that substance given to the subjects in a research project has become the scientific method. Anything less than this controlled method leaves question marks about the cause of any effect, and therefore, is unproven or unscientific.

The scientific method is great for certain things but it's not good for whole foods. Why? Because nature has combined many, many substances in every food to work synergistically in our bodies to promote vibrant health and longevity. So, over the last 100 years we have depended more and more on isolated substances that substitute for body functions rather than whole foods that regenerate your body.

Many times taking a supplement actually hurts our body. Taking hormones, for example, can weaken our body. Take a nutrient called Co-enzyme Q 10, whose job it is to move oxygen from the cell wall into the mitochondria of each cell in order to have proper metabolism. When oxygen is deficient, our metabolism is faulty and our energy level really drops. We get some Co-enzyme Q 10 in the food we eat, but more of it is produced in our liver by combining the lower Co Q's (Q9, Q8, Q7, etc.) to make Q10.

If a person has a deficiency of Co Q 10 and purchases a bottle of capsules, they may say how much more energy they have and how much better they feel. They will say, "I want to buy a case of that stuff!". However, supplying Co-enzyme Q 10 in supplemental form is substituting for the body. What we really want to do is cleanse and regenerate the liver so it can provide the body's requirements of Q 10 naturally. Do you see the difference? We are not doing ourselves a favor in the long run, when we take anything that substitutes for our body's normal functions. In fact, we may be doing a lot of harm, because generally, parts of the body that are not used grow weaker, not stronger, and we certainly don't need weaker body parts and functions!

While America was intoxicated with the scientific method, much of the "undeveloped" world thought that food—not drugs—made humans healthy. For thousands of years the Chinese have been at the forefront of such thought.

ESSENTIALS OF CHINESE HERBS

If we only look at these herbs as sources of new drugs, we will have missed the point.

A few years ago, medical researchers at the University of Texas collaborated with Chinese scientists on a research project. Their goal was to see if certain Chinese herbs could strengthen the body's immune system as ancient Chinese traditions said they could.

When they applied extracts from the herbs to cancer cells, they saw "a remarkable augmentative effect" on immunity—a strengthening, in other words. In fact, the treated cells ended up even stronger than normal. "We have something that works," the researchers told the Los Angeles Times. They also announced a ten-year project to develop the herbs, but the project has been canceled. No political support for it, the University of Texas said.

Even so, increasing numbers of scientists are beginning to look at Chinese herbs. As the research mounts, so does evidence showing that Chinese herbs work.

But there's a danger here. If we only look at these herbs as sources of new drugs, we will have missed the point. Chinese herbs represent a systematic view of the body and how it works. That way of thinking should not be separated from the herbs themselves. In fact, if we want to take full advantage of the herbs, we must begin by looking at the philosophy behind them.

First of all, the Chinese do not think of diseases as we know them. They think instead in terms of balance or imbalance. From the Chinese perspective, health is a pattern of harmony and balance, while ill health is a body out of balance.

The philosophy of regeneration says to feed your body back to health. Give the body all of the nutrients it needs, allow the body to get rid of wastes, and don't poison the body. Regeneration is treating the whole person, not their disease.

According to this Chinese philosophy, our body consists of paired opposites. These paired opposites depend on each other. They can't be separated. Their working together is what creates and sustains the whole.

Regeneration is treating the whole person, not just their disease.

The Chinese would word it differently, but to our scientific mind, the body includes the parasympathetic and sympathetic nervous systems. The parasympathetic nervous system gathers energy into the body; the sympathetic nervous system releases the gathered energy, or converts it into work. Put another way, the sympathetic nervous system spends energy—through moving, thinking, perceiving and communicating. The parasympathetic nervous system restores energy—through eating, drinking, sleeping and evacuating wastes. The rhythms of the body are nothing more than gathering and releasing, spending and restoring—and that balanced alternating is what keeps us going. We call it homeostasis.

From the Chinese point of view, we get sick when the rhythmic cycling gets out of balance. The Chinese don't spend much time studying and naming and treating diseases. They treat the entire person, restoring balance and health.

For example, the immune system consists of two general classes of cells: (1) those that attack and (2) those that inhibit, or shut off the attack.

Western physiologists now acknowledge that immune-system disorders come in two different varieties: (1) over-reactive disorders, characterized by too much attack, and (2) under-reactive disorders, characterized by too much suppression.

Allergies and autoimmune conditions are disorders that come from an overactive immune system.

Infections and tumors are disorders that come from an underactive immune system.

Immune System Too Strong	Immune System Too Weak
Allergies	Infections
Autoimmunity	Tumors

Immune System's Imbalances

Imbalances of this sort generally begin when particular body functions become weak. Chinese healers think of the body in terms of five major systems or functions.

The five major body systems are:

- Immune System
- Circulatory System
- Endocrine System
- Digestive System
- Respiratory System

This picture, however, is incomplete. To see things the way the Chinese see them, we've got to see them in motion. The theory of the five functions is above all, a study of motion.

So let's add motion to our picture. Envision "Energy flowing in a circle." These cycles of flowing energy connect the five basic functions in a loop. Energy flows from one to another until the flowing comes back to the beginning again, which completes the cycle, and the cycle starts again.

As the energy flows through this cycle, it builds, or becomes stronger, so that the functions promote or stimulate each other. As a consequence, the Chinese call this the "Promotion Cycle."

The Chinese also propose a second cycle. In this second cycle, the functions don't promote each other. They now inhibit, or suppress, or limit each other.

As the Promotion Cycle arouses the functions, so the Control Cycle calms them down. The two cycles operate in a partnership and the partnership keeps us in balance:

Since each function is always in motion, all of the functions are in motion. Viewed as a whole, however, the system appears to be in a state of equilibrium. This is the dynamic balance that traditional Chinese thought describes as the condition necessary for our normal growth, development and repair.

Homeostasis, Chinese Style

What would happen if the promotion cycle operated alone? Promotion would lead to more promotion, with each turn of the cycle exciting the functions further, and creating a vicious cycle. Eventually the system would burn itself out. These are the conditions that characterize illnesses of over activity.

What would happen if the control cycle operated by itself? Control would lead to more control, with each turn of the cycle depressing the functions. Eventually the system would stagnate. These are the conditions that characterize illnesses of under activity.

What happens when the two cycles operate in a balanced partnership? Each promotion is counterbalanced by a matching control, keeping activity and arousal constant. If some influence threatens the body's balance, the system counters it with a compensating shift in the opposite direction. Each cycle places limits on the other.

Although this Chinese explanation is thousands of years old, it's very close in concept to homeostasis, which refers to the body's ability to remain constant in the face of change. Homeostasis is the founding principle of modern physiology.

To our western scientific mind, traditional Chinese medicine's approach seems silly and all turned around. For over two thousand years the Chinese have placed the fruits, vegetables and herbs into three general groups, inferior, medium and superior. Inferior herbs would be poisonous or highly medicinal. Medium herbs would be somewhat medicinal. Superior herbs would be food, containing no chemicals that would force the body, but only nutrients that would feed the body.

To our Western scientific mind, traditional Chinese medicine's approach seems silly and all turned around.

If a Chinese healer were treating someone seriously ill, he would first treat the life threatening (considered secondary or non-causative) symptoms with inferior herbs. This is basically what western doctors do when they attack diseases with drugs.

Once the patient is out of danger, however, the Chinese healer would discontinue the inferior herbs and try to build strength in the patient using medium herbs. Once the patient is both stabilized and strengthened he would encourage regeneration, that is, the elimination of the underlying cause of the illness through the use of superior herbs. Superior herbs are, of course, food.

The Chinese believe that strong medicine is inferior. They also believe that life threatening symptoms are not the cause of the illness but the result of it, therefore secondary. So the Chinese first treat secondary symptoms with inferior herbs. Doesn't that sound backward? The Chinese also believe that overcoming the real cause of the illness can only be accomplished with superior herbs—FOOD. Food allows the body to balance itself and become healthy.

Drugs, of course, would be inferior to the Chinese. Most of the herbs we Americans can buy at the drug store or health food store would be medium herbs. Medium herbs override the body's control of itself more gently than drugs, but even this more gentle overriding can only achieve an artificial balance for the body.

Whole food concentrates should be made exclusively from "superior" herbs. They are food. The Chinese believe that certain foods feed certain functions of our body. If I were to ask you to name a food that fed a certain part of your body, you might be able to think of one or two—like a carrot for the eyes. For the most part, however, Westerners don't think of food for what body part or function it feeds. For thousands of years the Chinese have been researching and studying foods for how they affect the human body. And by the way, the Chinese have always used people in their studies, not rats. The Chinese deal with tens of thousands of herbs and foods, while we are lucky to know a couple of hundred.

Using this approach, the Chinese healers achieve a success rate of over 90 percent. They do not cure diseases with drugs, but strengthen bodies with foods. They do not heal bodies, they allow bodies to heal themselves.

As you know, this differs considerably from our western medical approach. We treat almost everything with strong medicine. And we satisfy ourselves with the kind of artificial, drug-sustained balance that the Chinese consider merely a first step. From the Chinese perspective, our healing system is naive and incomplete. From our perspective, of course, it is the Chinese system that is naive and incomplete.

The truth is, the Chinese have constructed their traditional healing model from centuries of scholarly research. And today, after two thousand years, when competent modern researchers test Chinese healing techniques, most of what they test turns out to work.

Applying the Principles

So how can we take advantage of this approach? By learning to use the food herbs of the Chinese. Food herbs are always safe. We can learn to use them by observing our own signs of imbalance. The step by which we build inner strength with foods is precisely what our own medical system is missing. In using food herbs, however, we must always remember this great advice: an ounce of prevention is worth a pound of cure.

The main purpose of Chinese food herbs is to build inner strength **before** we get sick. This is why Chinese healers were paid mainly for keeping people well.

Will these principles and practices work for us? Of course they will, and some day they'll become common and accepted. They won't replace our medical principles, for they address an entirely different goal.

Some might find it strange that an obviously Christian oriented book such as this would embrace a Chinese philosophy like regeneration. I'd certainly like to make clear that I don't embrace eastern religious philosophy. Regeneration, however, lines up with scriptural principles, whereas our own western philosophy based on the scientific model does not.

Ancient Chinese thought says that an unknown creator made mankind, and our bodies are capable of maintaining themselves. Science denies the existence of a creator and insists mankind evolved over millions of years from some single celled life form that was accidentally formed in some primeval swamp. Since there is no absolute, science thinks it has not only the right, but the obligation to "perfect" mankind, to help and to improve and to speed-up evolution. Under this philosophy medical intervention is okay, genetic engineering is okay, abortion is okay, assisted suicide is okay and euthanasia is okay.

Please don't misunderstand, I'm not saying that all science is bad. I am saying, however, that any system, any philosophy that denies God cannot be good.

Evolution has already been disproved many times and not just in faith by reading the creation story in Genesis (although that should be enough). For example, did you know that there are good, hard scientific facts that prove that man and dinosaurs lived contemporaneously? Human bones have been found with dinosaur bones? A human footprint has been found inside a dinosaur footprint? Read Job, Chapter 40 to find a description of a dinosaur.

The most convincing evidence against evolution, to my mind, is DNA. There are two primary reasons:

1. DNA is so incredibly complex and powerful. It stores the information about, and controls every aspect of our body. It is so small that it fits inside the nucleus of every cell in our body. The information storage capacity of DNA is so great that a single teaspoon of DNA could hold all the information on every species of organisms that ever lived, store all the information in every book that was ever written, with lots of room left over. Does that sound like an accident to you?

2. In order for DNA to make a copy of itself (as in growth) it makes an enzyme that controls the replication. Each is absolutely necessary for the other. That means the DNA code and the means of translating it had to appear separately but simultaneously if evolution is true. Even the contemplation of such an event happening is so ludicrous as to be incomprehensible.

WORDS TO KNOW

Synergy	Regeneration
Scientific Method	Sympathetic
Isolate	Parasympathetic
Synthetic	Homeostasis

SUMMARY

1. The human body is designed to eat food, not chemicals.
2. Our food today does not contain the nutrients it should.
3. Minerals, particularly, are deficient in our soils and therefore our food.
4. Healthy plants resist disease just as healthy bodies resist disease.
5. Food from healthy plants contain a huge variety of nutrients in just the right ratios that work synergistically to feed our bodies back to health.
6. Man-made nutrients do not have synergy and don't work nearly as well.
7. The scientific method is great for proving drugs, but can't work for food.
8. The philosophy of regeneration is nature's way to gain and maintain health.
9. For thousands of years the Chinese have used the philosophy of regeneration approach to health.
10. The scientific method as it is currently interpreted is based on evolution, not on creation.

21

UNDERSTANDING FAT MANAGEMENT

2 TIMOTHY 1:7

For God did not give us a spirit of timidity, but a spirit of power, of love and of self-discipline.

Being overweight is a sure sign that your body is malfunctioning and is one of the most common manifestations of malnutrition. Obesity is extremely wide spread; from young children to the elderly, it has become a major, national challenge. Like most problems, it is caused by ignoring correct principles. Also, when we try to correct the situation, we usually make matters worse by again following incorrect principles.

Strong flavors—an appeal to our carnality. We have 260 taste buds in our mouth. More often than not, these 260 taste buds dictate what nutrition our trillions of body cells receive. Talk about the minority ruling! We wouldn't put up with it in our government, would we? Strong flavors are almost always concentrated or refined or artificial. Flavors of fresh, whole foods tend to be much more subtle. In fact, they are sometimes considered bland when compared to the taste of concentrated, refined, artificial flavors. So what happens? Our appetite control mechanism of the feeling of fullness is overpowered by the sensual taste of the foods we are eating. When we eat fresh, whole, natural foods with their pleasant, yet more subtle flavors, we recognize the feeling of fullness and stop eating. Desserts are a case in point. If they weren't super sweet, we probably wouldn't eat them, because we are usually already full when we eat them.

One other very important point we need to make is the calorie-to-nutrition ratio. Fresh, whole, natural foods are loaded with nutrients and are relatively low in calories, while concentrated, refined, artificial foods are very high in calories and extremely low in nutrition. Sugar, for example, is 100% calories with NO nutrients! Junk food tastes great but has little or no nutritional value. We Americans have a tendency to eat far too much unhealthy food, thereby not leaving room for or having any inclination to include nutritious food in our diets. This creates a vicious cycle because we feel hungry if we have any nutritional deficiencies. So we wake up one morning, look in the mirror and say, "Yeah, I have to do something about this!"

Then most of us proceed to do exactly the wrong thing.

...DIET!!!

Only 3% of dieters succeed. That means 97% fail, most again and again. Diets are substitutes and do not regenerate. Dieters are trying to govern some of their body functions consciously rather than their bodies doing it unconsciously. When you diet you lose water, lean tissue and then, maybe, a little fat. For some time, researchers have known that severe calorie restriction forces the body to respond as if to starvation conditions. It conserves energy by lowering the metabolic pacemaker. The biological stage is set for regain on less food. As this dieting pattern continues, several bad things are likely to happen. Many studies have found that as weight is lost, both lean tissue and fat is lost, but regained weight is mostly fat. Dieting turns out to be the great fattener. Weight loss is fueled at cellular and hormonal levels. During a diet, fat cells shrink, they don't disappear. When normal eating is resumed, the fat cells don't just fill up with fat — they multiply, many times doubling in number. The new fat cells encourage your body to accumulate more fat. The next diet will be harder and failed diets, not just obesity, can sabotage health.

Many studies have found that as weight is lost, both lean tissue and fat is lost, but regained weight is mostly fat.

This feast-fast cycle itself can cause hypertension which leads to congestive heart failure, stroke, kidney disease and other things. Remember, the cause is not in the poundage alone but in the dieting pattern. The potent stress hormone, norepinephrine, is the link between body metabolism and blood pressure. When the brain signals danger, there are certain nerve cells that manufacture the "fight or flight" hormone norepinephrine. It in turn speeds heart-beat, constricts blood vessels and raises blood pressure. These nerve cells also respond to another kind of stress — over eating.

Weight is the least accurate measure of body fat content.

Dieting cycles can make norepinephrine producing nerve cells permanently hyperactive. A critical role in this disruption may be played at an area in the hypothalamus believed to be a brain control center for appetite, insulin levels and metabolism, as well as blood pressure. We must work WITH our biochemistry NOT at cross purposes to it! So again, NEVER DIET! It only leads to more fat and less health.

You don't have to look fat to be fat. Let's consider a 30 year old working mother who is slim and looks terrific in her clothes. She strictly watches her calories and participates in an aerobic workout at the local gym three times a week. Although she is managing to maintain her ideal weight, poor eating habits, bordering on a starvation diet, are actually making her fatter. Her metabolic rate has been suppressed, causing her slender body to catabolize its own muscle tissue while conserving its stores of fat. The result is a lower percentage of muscle and a higher percentage of body fat.

Weight is the least accurate measure of body fat content. That's why considering a person's weight at face value can give a very false impression.

BAD THINGS OFTEN HAPPEN WHEN YOU CUT CALORIES TOO MUCH.

The first thing that happens, when you cut calories drastically, occurs quickly. Within a matter of days, your metabolic rate will begin to slow down and your body will use up virtually all of its carbohydrate stores.

If a person also decides to limit carbohydrate intake as is so popular with many 'fad' diets, that person compounds the problem by cutting off her body's most accessible source of energy. She'll feel lethargic and unmotivated as well as hungry because her blood sugar level will be low. Oh, sure, the scales will say she's lost weight after a few days, but what she has really lost is mostly water. Here's how the vicious cycle works.

All the nutrients in whole food work together better than each part would separately.

Your body stores carbohydrates in the form of glycogen. Each gram of glycogen is stored in the body chemically bound to 3 grams of water, so when you drastically decrease your carbohydrate or calorie intake, liver and muscle glycogen stores fall, and the water that is bound to glycogen leaves the body. Since a gallon of water weighs about 8 pounds, you can eliminate a gallon of urine and you've lost 8 pounds.

That's a big loss, but not a good one. Depleting your carbohydrate energy stores, which come directly from muscle, amounts to a loss of lean body mass, leaving you with a greater percentage of body fat. On top of that, a low-carbohydrate diet (particularly one that leads to ketosis), can adversely impact your emotions and mental performance as well as make you feel terrible physically.

Some people live like this. Day in and day out they exist on near-starvation diets, drinking coffee and smoking cigarettes to gain a false energy boost from caffeine and nicotine. They may develop nutritional deficiencies, ending up with a body that has a low percentage of lean body mass and is subject to greater illness and osteoporosis later in life.

Unfortunately, when you decrease your metabolic rate, it can stay slowed down for a long time. That's why people who cut calories drastically or go on low-carb diets tend to rebound, that is, they hit the weight they want on the scale and say: "Okay, I've lost my weight. Now I can start eating normally again." The problem is, the body's suppressed metabolic rate suddenly has to deal with a lot more calories than it has adjusted itself to handle. That's where the rebound comes in and the pounds—especially fat—start piling back on faster than ever.

Any diet can lead to nutritional deficiencies. However, many experts believe that the low-carbohydrate diet will cause more of a metabolic slowdown than just restricting calories.

Your body reacts to the stress of low calorie dieting by secreting cortisol, a hormone than can increase the loss of lean body mass, especially when coupled with exercise. Cortisol impacts lean body mass by breaking it down and converting it to energy. It also depresses testosterone levels, signaling the body to store fat. A hormone found in both men and women, testosterone is central to fat metabolism so you want to avoid subjecting the body to this kind of dietary deprivation.

Experts believe that a low carbohydrate diet will cause more of a metabolic slowdown than just restricting calories.

According to federal government estimates, 58 million adults, or one-third of the adult population in the United States, are obese, which is defined in men as having 25% or more body fat and in women as having 30% or more body fat. Countless others just want to lose a little weight, so it's no surprise that any new weight-reducing "discovery" will get the attention of a public hungry for anti-obesity drugs.

You see, overweight people only have about 80% of the cellular energy of normal, healthy people. Because of this power shortage certain bodily functions are slowed down or eliminated. Since fat regulation takes a lot of energy and is not essential to life (like liver function or kidney function or brain function, etc.), it is one of the first processes to go. So we tend to store more fat, make less lean tissue, and have an even lower metabolism.

Most people remain pretty confused about the whole process. Diet gurus thrive on this confusion. Fat is big business and the hucksters know that they can continue to profit at the expense of an ever-fatter America by offering so-called revolutionary new products and programs that will make fat loss easy.

Actually, the answers to fat loss, and more importantly keeping it off, are crystal clear, but they don't come in a pill or a bottle. The key to building a great body is to change body composition by adding muscle, not just losing fat. Good nutrition is absolutely essential! Exercise is also extremely important. Resistance training is the best way to maintain or increase lean body mass, while moderate aerobic exercise is best for using up stored fat.

The key to building a great body is to change body composition by adding muscle, not just losing fat.

So, if we don't diet what do we do? Change your lifestyle and habits; 1) eat more fresh, whole foods and less processed, artificial foods, always checking for that calorie/nutrient ratio, 2) learn to handle stress... remember, being overweight for most people is very stressful in itself, 3) eat whole food concentrates specifically designed to raise cell energy and burn fat, 4) consider a moderate exercise program and increase your sunshine and fresh air, 5) periodically check your body composition for the percentage of fat and lean tissue... remember, the scales are a poor measure of progress!

Not all exercise is good for fat loss! Moderate, continuous, aerobic exercise is best. This is why. The fuel of your body is glucose. Your body can make fuel out of carbohydrate, protein or fat. It always uses up the carbohydrates first. So when we begin to exercise the body uses the glucose in the blood stream first. When that is used up, if we are still exercising, the body will convert the glycogen stored in our muscles and liver to glucose. To use the circulating glucose and stored glycogen usually takes between 15 to 20 minutes of continuous, moderate exercise. If our exercise is too strenuous, the body will convert protein (lean muscle mass) to fuel. But if we do everything right, that is, moderately exercise continuously for more than 20 minutes, the body will start to burn fat. Maintaining that level of exercise for 45 to 60 minutes is optimum for health when we are in shape. Most of us work up to that level slowly, while others cannot exercise until they lose some weight and gain some health. Of course, sunshine, fresh air and deep breathing all have very beneficial effects on weight management and health also.

WHOLE FOOD CONCENTRATES

These types of products are different! This type of program is in harmony with the theme of regeneration by working with the body to regenerate the body's fat maintenance process. It's a fat program that's actually good for the body. Most other diet programs focus on weight-loss with little regard to how it is accomplished. Most diet products use stimulants, laxatives and diuretics to artificially force the body to lose weight—usually water, and lean muscle tissue. This results in temporary weight loss and a feeling of hunger and fatigue. These synthetic diet pills are substitutes that threaten health, weaken the body's ability to control weight, and can create dependencies.

Synthetic diet pills are substitutes that threaten health, weaken the body's ability to control weight and can create dependencies.

In contrast, whole food concentrates emphasize Fat Management! They provide highly nutritious, whole foods in a concentrated form to fortify the body, helping to alleviate hunger and fatigue—the two most difficult problems to combat while establishing dietary control.

With these products your body will experience fat loss. They work with the body to burn fat for energy and flush excess fat out, through the body's elimination system. These whole food concentrates help the body build and regenerate the fat maintenance processes.

When you eat proper table foods and whole food concentrates, your body will receive the necessary nutrients needed to provide enough energy so it will choose to burn fat, resulting in permanent weight-loss. You have to take charge and be responsible for your own body!

There are concentrated herbal food formulas that support your body's efforts to be healthy as well as slender.

Certain formulas help the body speed up the process of linking lipids (fat) and protein into

Lipoproteins which are water soluble. This fat emulsification process is what gets fat out of storage and makes it available to be burned as fuel.

Some formulas are thermogenic. That is, they nourish and support your body's natural ability to convert stored fat into energy. Remember, they are food, not forcers! They have no detrimental side effects. Other thermogenic products like ephedra, mahuang and ephedrine force fat metabolism at the expense of overall health. Severe health-robbing side effects have been the rule with most weight loss systems.

This fat emulsification process is what gets fat out of storage and makes it available to be burned as fuel.

There is an herb beverage that feeds the restorative functions of our body. One of its many traits is its ability to carry free fat (fat in the bloodstream) out of the body through urination. That's a lot better than having it stored in the adipose tissue!

There is a highly nutritious bar that contains eight grams of fiber. Fiber binds with fat in the digestive tract and carries it out with the feces. Most Americans eat just 30 to 35% of the recommended amount of dietary fiber. One bar goes a long way in making up this deficit.

EATING ICE CAN HELP YOU LOSE WEIGHT...

Think about it—a very pleasant way to get your needed water intake while at the same time using up 200 to 300 extra calories every week. Here is the math. It takes 80 calories to heat 2 quarts of water from 32° to 98.6°. I haven't seen any research on it but you can't deny the math. Of course, you would want to use distilled water to make your ice and crush it before you eat it. It would mean a little preparation and being near a freezer. You might get laughed at by your family or your fellow workers. Like any good fat loss program, it is not a quick fix. However, it can be a healthy and effective tool to add to your fat management toolbox.

The combination of an intelligent menu and the whole food concentrates will begin to remove excess fat, decrease inches, while increasing energy, building muscle tone and restoring vital health.

The intelligent menu would cut way down on fat in all forms; all pork, fatty red meats, all fried foods, vegetable oil in margarine, baked goods, salad dressings, etc.; also refined sugar and white flour products should be restricted, i.e.: ice cream, sodas, candy, baked goods of all kinds; pies, cakes, bread and rolls made with white flour, crackers, breakfast cereals and most processed, refined foods that come out of a can or a box. In other words, eat much more fresh agricultural products and eat whole food concentrates for maximum results.

The intelligent menu would cut way down on fat in all forms.

Luke 21:34 says, "Be careful, or your hearts will be weighted down with dissipation, drunkenness and anxieties of life, and that day will close on you unexpectedly like a trap." The word dissipation means to over eat, gluttony, to indulge in pleasure to the point of harming oneself. And "that day" is when Christ returns and the future aspect of God's kingdom is inaugurated. In other words, in the last days, people will be given to worry and overindulgence. Could it be these very days we are living in?

WORKSHEET 1

DAILY CALORIE NEEDS

APPROXIMATE YOUR CALORIE MAINTENANCE LEVEL (CML) AS FOLLOWS:

A. Your approximate ideal weight in front of the zero (A) ____________0

Example: 120 lbs. (A) 1200

B. Take 25% of A (Divide A by 4) = (B) ____________

Example: 1200 ÷ 4 = (B) 300

C. Add A to B — A+B= ____________

Your CML

Example 1200 + 300 = 1500
(A) (B) CML

PART 2

Calculate how many grams of carbohydrates, protein and fat you should eat daily.

Your CML ____________		____________	
A. Carbohydrates:	CML X .70 =	____________	Carb calories
	Divided by 4 =	____________	grams Carbs
B. Protein:	CML X .15 =	____________	Protein calories
	Divided by 4 =	____________	grams Protein
C. Fat:	CML X .15 =	____________	Fat calories
	Divided by 9 =	____________	grams Fat

EXAMPLE: *1500 X .70 = 1050 . . . Divided by 4 = 262 grams of Carbs*

1500 X .15 = 225 . . . Divided by 4 = 56 grams of Protein

1500 X .15 = 225 . . . Divided by 9 = 25 grams of Fat

FAT ITEMS

FOODS:	FAT GRAMS:
3 CHOCOLATE SANDWICH COOKIES	6 Grams
3 PATS OF BUTTER	12 Grams
8 OZ. OF WHOLE MILK	8.15 Grams
1 TBSP. COOKING OIL	13.5 Grams
1 MEDIUM ORDER OF FRENCH FRIES	17 Grams
1 FAST FOOD TACO	11 Grams
1 SLICE OF AMERICAN CHEESE	7 Grams
1 TBSP. ITALIAN SALAD DRESSING	7 Grams
1/4 POUND OF HAMBURGER	23 Grams
1 APPLE	0 Grams
1 WATERMELON	0 Grams
1 CUP OF GREEN BEANS	0 Grams
1 HEAD OF LETTUCE	0 Grams

FIBER IN FOODS

11 Carrots	8 Grams fiber
7.5 Cups Green Beans	8 Grams fiber
13 Tomatoes	8 Grams fiber
12.5 Small Naval Oranges	8 Grams fiber
1.5 Pineapples	8 Grams fiber
1 Pound Brussels Sprouts	8 Grams fiber
1 Head Cauliflower	8 Grams fiber
5.5 Pounds Cantaloupe	8 Grams fiber
17.5 Small Bananas	8 Grams fiber

WORDS TO KNOW

Norepinephrine

Glycogen

Cortisol

SUMMARY

1. Being over-fat is a sure sign of malnutrition.
2. Strong flavors are an appeal to our carnality.
3. NEVER DIET!
4. Dieting cycles cause imbalances.
5. Low carbohydrate diets are especially bad.
6. There is no magic pill.
7. Whole food concentrates can help.

22

EXERCISE

1 TIMOTHY 4:8

For physical training is of some value, but godliness has value for all things, holding promise for both the present life and the life to come.

We need more oxygen more often than anything else. We need oxygen more than water, more than food, more than any nutrient. And we need it in every cell of our body. Oxygen is essential to the process of ionization, or the breaking down of food into the nutrients suitable for our body's use. We need oxygen to burn glucose and produce energy from metabolism. Without sufficient oxygen in our bloodstream our cells literally suffocate. Our brain suffers first because it requires about three times more oxygen than most other organs and tissues.

It should come as no surprise to you that the great majority of the oxygen we receive comes by way of our lungs, through the function we know as breathing. (We get some oxygen through our skin). It might surprise you, however, to learn that the average American usually only uses about one-half of their lungs. The way you use your lungs has a very great impact on your health, your looks, the way you feel and your very life span! So the way we breathe is hugely important. We need to use our full lung capacity all the time or we are robbing our body, particularly our brain, of needed oxygen with dire consequences. Example—Dr. Philip Rice, M.D., a morphologist who has worked for years with delinquent children, estimates that over half of the delinquency in minors can be attributed to oxygen starvation.

The first thing we need to understand is the mechanism by which the oxygen is distributed to every cell in the body—the cardiovascular system. The oxygen is carried in your bloodstream by the red blood corpuscles. There are millions of these cells in every drop of blood. There are about 100,000 miles of blood vessels in the average individual filled with six to eight quarts of blood. During rest the blood makes about one round trip per minute, but during activity it can make as many as eight or nine round trips per minute to supply the needed fuel and oxygen for energy, and the removal of waste products. The human heart is divided into two halves, each half having two pumping chambers. The right side of the heart pumps the blood to the lungs, the left side pumps the blood to the rest of the body. So there are really two circulation systems. The lesser circulation, as it is called, goes from the heart to the lungs and back. This is vital so that waste products like carbon dioxide can be discharged and so the life-giving oxygen can be absorbed.

Shallow breathers are actually poisoning themselves, torturing their cells, and committing slow suicide; all for the lack of vital oxygen.

The lungs are very large but very delicate organs. If you could spread your lungs out, they would cover about two tennis courts. They are composed of some 800 million alveoli or air sacs, made of elastic tissue, that expand and contract like tiny balloons. As the blood returns from feeding the cells of the body, it has no oxygen left in it, but it is loaded with toxic waste products. This blood is channeled through all the capillaries of our lungs, but only the air sacs with air in them are of any use. The blood that passes through the capillaries of empty air sacs cannot get rid of its carbon dioxide wastes and cannot pick up any oxygen. So instead of carrying a full quota of oxygen back to the cells of the body, the blood returns with a mixture of fresh oxygen and a residue of toxic wastes. As this process continues the proportion of waste products in the blood stream increases. And remember, the average American only uses one-half of his lungs.

Loaded with poisonous wastes, the blood cannot supply the amount of oxygen needed by the cells nor can it carry the necessary nourishment from food. The breaking down of food molecules is impaired while all body functions are slowed down. The organs of elimination are overworked and underfed. So these toxic wastes are deposited in heavy mucous in our sinus cavities, bronchial tubes and lungs, and we think we have another cold or more allergies. Shallow breathers are actually poisoning themselves, torturing their cells, and committing slow suicide; all for the lack of vital oxygen. Your lungs are designed to hold between six and ten pints of air. Fill them up—use them all!

When the sternum is carried high and the rib cage expanded, the lungs are in position to be filled with air.

The main muscle that does our breathing is called the diaphragm. The diaphragm is a dome-shaped sheet of muscle that separates the thoracic (chest) cavity containing the heart and lungs, from the abdominal cavity housing the other organs. As the diaphragm works it expands the chest cavity drawing air into the lungs. It also expands the abdominal cavity exercising the muscles and organs. This expansion and relaxation of the diaphragm has a beneficial effect on the organs of the abdomen. It provides a massage for the liver, stomach, intestines, kidneys, gall bladder, spleen and pancreas—stimulating the flow of blood through these vital organs. The solar plexus is located in the center of the diaphragm, the more circulation received by the solar plexus, the greater the nerve energy going to your organs.

Posture is extremely important! When you slump you squeeze your lungs and seriously hamper the operation of your diaphragm, making yourself a shallow breather. You also impair circulation and thereby hamper most vital functions and become fatigued. Crossing your legs, all tight clothing or anything that restricts circulation is to be avoided. There is no feeling of well-being as great as when every cell in your body is filled with life-giving oxygen.

Have you ever experienced a "stitch" in your side after a little forced exercise? You had just discovered a portion of unused lung. The unused air sacs of your lungs have a tendency to collapse upon themselves and stick together. The sharp pain is the air forcing them apart again. Most of us need to learn to breathe properly so the following are several exercises that will help.

When the sternum is carried high and the rib cage expanded, the lungs are in position to be filled with air. The uplifted diaphragm also draws into position the prolapsed organs of the abdomen. For an exercise that strengthens this posture, stand with heels and toes together. Raise both hands high over your head while also rising on your tiptoes—stretch. Repeat ten times. Stretching is a great form of health building, almost all animals do it.

Next, with your arms at your sides, draw up the contents of your abdomen as though everything were up in the chest cavity. Then push everything down into your protruding belly. Repeat 10 times. Now do the same exercise but this time with your arms over your head and walking on your toes. Ten times. If you feel dizzy, stop and rest. You may need to start with a few repetitions and build up to 10.

Finally, use this last exercise to oxygenate the brain and pituitary gland. Stand erect, feet about 18 inches apart, arms relaxed at your sides. Raise your hands overhead. Now bend forward as far as possible, keeping the knees bent, at the same time exhaling through the mouth—push every bit of air out of your lungs. Now, slowly inhale as you start upright. As you do this bring your arms upward to the overhead position. Repeat 10 times.

THE BENEFITS OF EXERCISE

Every day the list gets longer! Everyone knows that exercise is good for you. (Some people are tired of hearing about it, and wish the health nuts would just leave them alone!) But why it's good is less understood. Even the people who are already exercising probably don't realize all the good things they're doing, so we're going to give you a quick rundown of the most important ones.

First, we should define what we mean by exercise. We're talking about aerobic exercise, the kind that gets you moving vigorously enough to speed up your heartbeat for at least 20 minutes at a time, preferably 30 to 45 minutes, at least three times a week. Running, walking briskly, cycling, swimming, skating and aerobic dancing are some examples.

A good workout relieves stress and does it better than a cigarette or martini.

IMMEDIATE BENEFITS

- **Relieves tension.** Feeling depressed, uptight, or angry? A good workout gets rid of your stress—and does a better job of it than a cigarette or a double martini.
- **Improves sleep.** Not only does vigorous exercise help you fall asleep faster, you sleep sounder, so you get more 'good' from each hour you're asleep.
- **Reduces appetite.** Really! Many people think it's the other way around, but exercise is actually an appetite depressant. That's one reason it's best to exercise before meals, rather than after.
- **Clears the mind.** When you go for a three-mile jog or brisk walk, your mind tends to wander. When your mind wanders, it often comes up with surprisingly brilliant thoughts.
- **Promotes companionship.** A lot of people are doing all sorts of exercise these days. If you exercise, you're likely to find someone who'll join you.
- **It's fun.** If the exercise you choose is something you like to do, you're more likely to stick with it. And the more you do it, the more fun it will be.

LONG-TERM BENEFITS

- **Strengthens the heart.** The more you exercise, the more blood your heart can pump with each beat. So it doesn't have to beat as often, which is good.
- **Improves circulation.** As you exercise, your body actually develops additional capillaries—the tiny blood vessels that deliver oxygen to the cells. The more capillaries, the more oxygen gets to the cells which is also good.

Exercises like jogging, walking and dancing help keep bones strong.

- **Fat control.** Besides reducing appetite, exercise increases metabolism, which helps you burn more calories even when you're not exercising.
- **Increases HDL.** HDL is a kind of protein in the blood that scientists have found helps remove harmful buildups of cholesterol in the blood vessels. People who exercise have more HDL than inactive people.
- **Eases hypertension.** People who get regular aerobic exercise have lower blood pressure than people who don't. And people who have high blood pressure can bring it down by exercising.
- **Helps treat diabetes.** Exercise increases a person's sensitivity to insulin. For diabetics, this means more effective treatment of their disease with less need for insulin.
- **Strengthens bones.** A leading cause of disability among people over 50 is fractures caused by gradually weakening bones. Exercises like jogging, walking and dancing help keep bones strong.
- **Trims the figure.** Where there may have been fat, exercise creates muscles. Where there may have been unwanted bulges and unflattering flabbiness, exercise brings sleek, lean, firm profiles.

- **Makes you feel alive.** There's nothing like a good stiff workout to make you feel alert and alive. And it's a feeling that lasts long after you've stopped sweating.

The Vital Warm-up and Cool-down

Don't forget to spend five minutes preparing for and recovering from exercise.

Some people find it hard enough to psych themselves up to exercise, let alone for some warm-up work beforehand and cool-down afterwards. But it's worth the effort. The pre and post exercise routines are the best way to keep your exercise safe and injury-free.

To understand the importance of the warm-up, consider what your body is like before you get started exercising. Chances are you've been sitting somewhere for a while—either at a desk, on a sofa, or driving a car. Your heart is at its resting pulse rate. Your muscles are at rest.

To go from that state to a full-demand level of activity in a few seconds is simply more than many bodies can handle without breaking down. You're asking the heart to more than double its rate, while pumping larger volumes with each beat at the same time. And you're asking cold, stiff muscles to suddenly begin flexing and extending to their full extent.

A lot of times, the body's ability to absorb punishment will prevent injury under this kind of assault. But sooner or later, something has to give. Most torn muscles are the result of failure to warm up. It's much more sensible to put in a few minutes of gentle warm-up to stay out of trouble.

A typical warm-up session might consist of some stretching exercises, with particular emphasis on those muscles that you'll be using the most during exercise, followed by some easy calisthenics, brisk walking, or easy jogging. Whatever you do, the routine should have the dual effect of gently stretching your leg, back and arm muscles and accelerating your heart rate.

Many exercisers who reluctantly perform their warm-ups before hitting the road still find it too much bother to cool down afterwards. But that five-minute finale is just as important as the prelude. One study found that more than half of all exercise-related fatalities occurred in the few minutes after exercise, to people who didn't cool down.

Again, it helps to picture what you're asking of your body. At the end of a strenuous workout, your heart is pumping 150 or so times a minute to supply your body with its increased need for oxygen. Your muscles are warm, loose, and full of the "exhaust" products of their hard work, mainly lactic acid.

If you stop suddenly, and sit or lie down, your body still needs a greater-than-normal supply of blood for a while, but the muscle contractions that have been giving the heart some assistance are now quiet and the heart has to do everything by itself. Most of the time, it will. Occasionally, the heart simply can't handle the unassisted load and the result could be a heart attack.

The other reason for cooling down is to give those muscles a chance to work off the lactic acid, which otherwise could cause cramps later on. Some exercise specialists say the stretch you do after exercise is even more important than the one before.

A cool-down routine can be pretty much the same as the warm-up—gentle, smooth, easy activity, something that keeps the muscles moving and brings the heartbeat back down gradually.

If you have been leaving off these vital portions of your exercise routine, try to incorporate them next time. See if you don't notice a better workout and a lot less stiffness and soreness the next few days.

Man or beast, male or female, we all age the same way. Muscles atrophy, that is, shrink in size and strength as the fat layer grows.

Without a regimented and active exercise program the average American after the age of 35 loses $1/2$ pound of muscle and gains $1\frac{1}{2}$ pounds of fat each year. Not only do we gain weight, we shift from muscle weight to fat weight. As we age—young and strong gives way to old and fat.

You don't have to kill yourself to get the benefits of exercise. With some things in life, the more the better. But with others, there's a point at which you can start doing more harm than good. Exercise fits that category.

Without a regimented and active exercise program, the average American, after the age of 35, loses ½ pound of muscle and gains 1½ pounds of fat each year.

People exercise for many reasons, but certainly one of the biggest is the fear of heart disease. In the beginning of the running movement, a myth was born that anyone who could run a marathon would be immune to a heart attack. That myth has been shattered, most notably by the death, after running, of author Jim Fixx, a man who had competed in many marathons. Fixx apparently ignored some warning signs of heart trouble, and it cost him his life. Running, and other forms of exercise, can do a lot of good, but they aren't the route to immortality.

What the experts are discovering is that there's an optimal level of heart-strengthening exercise and when you go much beyond that, the stress you put on your body damages it more than the benefits help it. Among the risks that increase: joint injuries, stress fractures, and various strains and sprains. The optimal level is roughly equivalent to burning 2,000 calories per week.

People who exercise regularly at the 2,000 calorie level have been found to reduce their death rate by as much as a third compared to those who don't exercise at all. Those who exercise more than 2,000 calories worth gain some added protection, but not much. Beyond 3,500 calories a week the net health benefits start decreasing.

What does 2,000 calories mean in terms of actual exercise? It depends on several factors, including your weight, the intensity of the exercise, and your skill at performing the exercise. Here are some representative exercise prescriptions that would burn the 2,000 calories each week. These figures are based on performing the exercise four times per week in order to reach the 2,000 calorie total.

- For someone who weighs 120 pounds, 6 miles of jogging four times a week is all you need. For a 170 pounder, 4 miles is enough. (The heavier you are, the more energy it takes to perform the same exercise).
- If jogging isn't your style, briskly walking the same number of miles burns the same number of calories.
- Swimming 2,500 yards (for a 120 pound person) or 1,700 yards (170 pounds).
- Bicycling 13 miles (120 pounds) or 9 miles (170 pounds).
- 65 minutes of aerobic dancing (120 pounds), or 45 minutes (170 pounds).

The optimal exercise level is roughly equivalent to burning 2,000 calories per week.

Of course, you can stay in reasonably good shape doing less exercise than this. But these regimens will give you the optimum level of cardiovascular fitness.

In addition to the heart-strengthening effect, this 2,000-calorie-per-week program gives you, you'll be helping yourself take off unwanted fat. Someone who burned an extra 2,000 calories a week, and didn't change the amount of food eaten, would lose about 30 pounds in one year.

Walking just may be the perfect exercise; it's certainly the simplest. Walking is deceptive. Since it's so easy, it's hard to believe that it could be that good for you. But walking is almost as good a conditioner as running. It will burn up nearly as many calories per mile—about 100. It strengthens the heart, lowers blood pressure and resting pulse rate, increases muscle tone, reduces blood cholesterol levels, and relieves stress.

Walking is something everyone knows how to do. You don't need any special equipment, other than a good pair of walking shoes. Unlike running and other strenuous activities, walking poses almost no risk of injury. And walking is convenient—you can walk anywhere, anytime, alone or with a crowd.

REST

Rest means repose, freedom from activity, quiet, tranquil. It means peace of mind and spirit. It means an absence of anxiety or worry and it means to refresh yourself. To rest means to allow free circulation of blood to the entire body, so don't wear anything tight or lie on your arm and cut off the blood supply. The art of resting is something that most of us must acquire and do deliberately. Of course, tobacco, drugs, coffee, tea, alcohol and cola drinks all jangle the nerves in some way and prevent complete rest and relaxation.

The art of resting is something that many of us must acquire and do deliberately.

Sleep is different from rest. You can rest without sleeping and sleep without resting. One bad habit in modern America is the midnight snack. You cannot get a good night's sleep if you overload your stomach.

A healthy adolescent or adult usually doesn't suffer any harm from occasionally missing a few hours' sleep. The traditional notion that it is necessary to sleep eight hours each night has no basis, in fact. We vary a great deal in sleep requirements, some functioning quite nicely on five hours sleep, while others require eight or nine hours. But every one of us needs rest and sleep if we are to be healthy. Our body's and mind's ability to work is restored during restful sleep. Many physical repairs of the body occur only during sleep. And, although we don't know why, people who are deprived of dreaming are adversely affected physically, mentally and emotionally.

You can rest without sleeping and sleep without resting.

Finally, I would like to mention that even God rested. Genesis 2:2, "By the seventh day God had finished the work He had been doing; so on the seventh day He rested from all His work."

WORDS TO KNOW

Alveoli

Diaphragm

Solar Plexus

Atrophy

SUMMARY

1. We need more oxygen more consistently than any other nutrient.
2. Most people only use about $\frac{1}{2}$ of their lung capacity.
3. Deep breathing and exercise are extremely beneficial to every organ of your body.
4. Warming up before and cooling down afterward are very important to the success of an exercise program.
5. The optimum amount of exercise seems to be burning between 2,000 and 3,500 calories per week.
6. Resting and sleeping are two different things and both are essential to good health.

23

LIGHT AND SUNSHINE

Down through history sunlight has been revered for its life-giving and healing powers. Observations were made and records kept that showed the sun to be a positive factor in health. In 1877 Downes and Blunt discovered that sunlight destroyed bacteria. In 1903 Niels Finsen won the Nobel Prize for treating tuberculosis with ultraviolet light. Many other studies have revealed the potent, beneficial and multifaceted effects of sunlight on the human body. Things like:

GENESIS 1:3-4

And God said, "Let there be light," and there was light. God saw that the light was good.

1. Improves electrocardiogram
2. Lowers blood pressure
3. Lowers resting heart rate
4. Increases cardiac output
5. Lowers blood cholesterol
6. Increases glycogen stores in the liver
7. Decreases blood sugar levels
8. Increases energy, endurance and muscular strength
9. Increases melatonin production
10. Lowers CAMP (cyclic adenasine monophosphate)
11. Strengthens the immune system

12. Increases oxygen carrying capacity of blood
13. Increases tolerance to stress
14. Increases sex hormones
15. Increases resistance to infections

Sunlight has been found to have much the same effect on the body as exercise.

Even with all of these known benefits of sunlight, it is no longer used therapeutically. In fact, sunlight is now looked on as a threat mainly because of the fear of skin cancer. Ever since Domagk won the Nobel Prize in 1939 for treating bacterial infections with drugs, the pharmacologic dominance in medical therapy has increased. Even so, let's examine some of the many benefits of sunlight.

We all know that a program of endurance exercises greatly increases the fitness of the individual. This results in a much higher level of energy for better performance in work or play and also allows us to endure stress much better. This general improvement in physical condition is caused by better circulation and its ability to carry life-giving oxygen into the tissues. Our body becomes more efficient in many ways. The resting heart rate decreases, the respiratory rate decreases and so does lactic acid. Our lungs absorb more oxygen, our blood carries more oxygen and our muscle cells utilize more oxygen than before.

Sunlight, has been found to have much the same effect on the body as exercise. The mechanism may not be the same as that used by exercise, but they both increase the oxygen in the tissues. Just think of the multiplied benefits if you exercised in the sunshine and fresh air! The ancient Greeks, who worshiped the beauty of the well-formed body, took this idea to the ultimate—exercising nude on a warm sandy beach. This was especially beneficial for males because of the increased testosterone production. Testosterone is that hormone responsible for muscular development. In fact, studies have shown that combined sunlight and exercise worked twice as well as exercise alone in improving electrocardiograms of recovering heart attack victims. Maybe that is why some of the most popular TV exercise shows take place on the beach. Other studies have proven that exercise and sunlight or a combination of both, lowers high blood pressure and high blood sugar levels, as well as increasing the output of blood from the heart.

The effect of sunlight on blood sugar metabolism is like that of insulin. It apparently facilitates the absorption of glucose into the cells for "burning" or into glycogen (stored carbohydrates) which is stored in the liver and muscles.

As we have already pointed out in another chapter, cholesterol is not the villain that many medical authorities claim it to be. In fact, it is the raw material out of which the body makes many valuable substances, such as bile salts, sex hormones (progesterone, estrone, estradiol, testosterone and osterone), Vitamin D, cortisone and aldosterone. Sunlight striking the exposed skin lowers total cholesterol. The concentration of cholesterol is higher in our skin than other organs. Sunshine changes this cholesterol into a previtamin D substance and then body heat changes it into Vitamin D in about 24 hours. In the meantime, other hormones are made from the previtamin D.

Recently it has been revealed that Vitamin D is not as much a vitamin as it is a hormone, and hormones are regulated by delicate balances of several glands that work in concert. Dietary supplementation of hormones disturb this balance and cause lots of problems. For many years now the commercial food industry has been responsible for the prolific supplementation of Vitamin D hormone in many foods; including baby foods, imitation dairy products, many beverages, sauces, breakfast cereals, margarine, macaroni, noodles, farina, flour and of course, milk.

It has been known for years that dietary Vitamin D causes heart attacks in experimental animals. Now scientists at New York University have shown that some heart attacks are triggered by loss of magnesium from the heart tissue and that dietary Vitamin D causes a magnesium deficiency in the heart. Also, Vitamin D hormone has been identified as an angiotoxic substance, that is, a substance that irritates the lining of blood vessels. This damage to the arteries is definitely a step in the development of atherosclerosis.

Every attempt should be made to restrict your intake of processed foods supplemented with vitamin D

Every attempt should be made to restrict your intake of processed foods supplemented with Vitamin D, and rely on the natural production within your body produced by sunlighting the skin.

Of all the benefits sunshine gives us, one of the most important is its effect on infectious diseases. This happens for two reasons. Sunlight kills germs. Sunlight strengthens the immune system. During the latter part of the 1800's, and up to 1939, sunlight therapy was the most effective for most infectious diseases including anthrax bacillus, coccobacillus, strep, tubercle bacillus, cholera bacillus, staph, colon bacillus, and dysentery bacillus. Then in 1938 penicillin was discovered and the era of antibiotics and drug therapy began. This event signed the death warrant to sunlight therapy. After more than 50 years of antibiotics, germs are stronger and people are weaker, to the extent that we may witness the development of a new microbial strain that could cause a world-wide pandemic, against which all the wonder drugs of modern science would be futile.

Our skin is an effective barrier against most germs. Exposure to sunlight aids the skin by killing pathogens on the surface. Even the sweat has an acidity which is very unfavorable to germs. Sunlight also changes skin oils into bacteriocidal agents and even the vapors rising from these oils kill bacteria. For these reasons acne can be treated by sunlight.

If pathogens get through the skin or mucous membrane the body's defense systems are triggered. The greatest lines of defense against invading germs is found in the circulatory system and the lymphatic system.

Usually the first cell to meet an invader is a macrophage. It "eats" the germ, analyzes it, and determines its make up. It passes this information to white blood cells called lymphocytes which either attack the invading germs or make antibodies—one works in the bloodstream and the other works in the cell. Lymphocytes work within the cells by making chemicals that either destroy the germ or signal for reinforcements. The help that comes is the macrophage which "eat" the germs. Antibodies or gamma globulins work in the blood to neutralize the germs by combining with them or marking the germ to be eaten by white blood cells. Studies have proven that sunlight increases the number and strength of lymphocytes and antibodies. Increased lymphocytes and gamma globulins, obviously enhance our ability to fight all kinds of disease.

Studies have proven that sunlight increases the number and strength of lymphocytes and antibodies.

Lymphocytes also produce a substance called interferon. Interferon has the ability to stop the reproduction of viruses. It is even effective against several different kinds of cancer including carcinoma, sarcoma, and leukemia. Other viral infections like hepatitis, herpes simplex, herpes zoster, chicken pox, and the common cold are improved by interferon. Again, sunlight is a great stimulus for increased lymphocyte production and thereby, more interferon.

Other white blood cells called phagocytes have the ability to eat foreign substances. The most common of the phagocytes are neutrophils. They are found in large numbers at the site of any infection or injury. After an injury neutrophils respond in minutes and in less than two hours are present in huge numbers. Ultraviolet waves, particularly from sunlight, stimulate the neutrophils to eat germs more rapidly, up to twice as many, twice as fast.

Since sunlight is able to eliminate bacteria from air, water and skin, and also strengthens our immune system, it would follow that persons that sunbathe regularly would develop fewer illnesses and this is exactly what happens. A word of caution is necessary here. Never get too much sun or get it too fast. Forty-five minutes a day is ideal. More than this, particularly in warmer climates in the middle of the day is too much. For those sun bathers who are looking for an excuse to bake in the sun, this discussion is NOT that excuse. Getting too much sun or getting it too quickly is definitely detrimental!

There is a substance found in most cells, especially immune cells like lymphocytes, whose chemical name is cyclic adenosine monophosphate. We will simply call it CAMP. As CAMP increases in lymphocytes and other immune cells, they become unable to function properly and will not destroy bacteria, cancer cells, etc. In other words CAMP inhibits our immune system. The things that stimulate the production of CAMP are polyunsaturated fats, adrenalin caused by stress, coffee, tea and chocolate.

For those sun bathers who are looking for an excuse to bake in the sun, this discussion is NOT that excuse.

Fortunately, CAMP is sensitive to light and easily destroyed by it. Sunlight penetrates deep into the body and lowers the level of CAMP. This reduction of CAMP produces a relaxing effect on the nervous system. Just as caffeine stimulates the nervous system by increasing CAMP, so sunlight relaxes us by decreasing CAMP.

All air is not created equal. Air is made up of both positively and negatively charged ions. Good fresh outdoor air is usually about 45% negative, 55% positive. All heating and cooling units change negative ions into positive ions. As positive ions increase and negative ions decrease, we feel such adverse effects as headache, fatigue, dizziness, etc. Conversely, negatively charged air produces a feeling of well-being and exhilaration. It has been shown that negative air inhibits the growth of cancer. Living and working indoors leaves us vulnerable to stress because positive air depresses the adrenal glands to make hormones that protect us. Negatively charged air increases the mucous flow in the respiratory system. This is important because germs don't have time to proliferate and cause an illness like bronchitis or pneumonia. Yes, you guessed it! Sunlight produces negatively charged air.

Sunlight helps in weight management by stimulating the thyroid gland and by increasing muscle tone—both burn more calories.

Sunlight has the ability to speed up the elimination of toxic agents from our body, but too much sunshine (burning) does not produce this effect. Tests have been run on such noxious chemicals as lead, mercury, fluoride, pesticides, carbon tetrachloride, etc. Animals given sunlight treatments eliminated these chemicals 10 to 20 times as fast as animals kept indoors. The ultraviolet light increases enzymes that metabolize toxic chemicals and remove them.

Sunlight is very helpful in overcoming jaundice, arthritis, ulcers, gout, psoriasis, acne and obesity. It helps in weight management by stimulating the thyroid gland and by increasing muscle tone—both burn more calories.

Just a few precautions will take all the danger out of sunbathing. First of all, don't get burned. Long exposures to the midday sun should be avoided. Because sunlight increases free radical formation, don't eat refined polyunsaturated fat. This is where a lot of free radicals come from. Get plenty of antioxidants in your diet. Antioxidants prohibit free radical formation. Avoid suntan oils and lotions. They are absorbed into the skin and changed into free radicals. Sunscreens limit the benefits received. Moderate exposure is the way to control burning, not oils and screens.

Just because it is a cloudy day doesn't mean we can't receive great benefits from being outdoors. The air is much more negatively charged and 80% of the ultraviolet waves, which are so helpful, penetrate even totally overcast skies. So get outside and do something. Your body will be glad you did!

WORDS TO KNOW

Hormones

Angiotoxic

Antibiotics

Pandemic

Lymphocytes

CAMP (Cyclic Adenosine Monophosphate)

Ions

Ultraviolet

SUMMARY

1. Light and sunshine provide a multitude of health benefits to the human body.
2. Sunlight has been found to have much the same effect on the body as exercise.
3. Sunlight changes cholesterol into Vitamin D.
4. Sunlight kills germs and strengthens the immune system to help fight infectious diseases.
5. Outdoor air is better for us than indoor air.
6. Sunlight helps eliminate toxins from the body.

CONCLUSION

Many of us are looking for a quick, easy solution to our problems. We're searching for that magic pill, that miracle cure. Most of you probably think I'm going to tell you that there is no magic pill or miracle cure. Well, you're wrong. There is one miracle that is sufficient for every human problem. That miracle, of course, is God sending His Son, Jesus Christ to pay the penalty for our transgressions and shortcomings, so that those who accept His free gift of salvation can live eternally with Him in perfect health. Perhaps the most famous verse in the whole Bible is John 3:16. Read it again (or for the first time) and rejoice in it.

ECCLESIASTES 12:13

Now all has been heard; here is the conclusion of the matter: Fear God and keep His commandments, for this is the whole duty of man

As for our physical health in this present world, alas, there is no magic pill. The best we can do is to try to do things God's way, by following the instructions He has given us.

Our physical health, good or bad, is the result of the aggregate effect of everything we allow to enter into us. Let's consider some of those things:

Air Do you have good posture? Do you breathe deeply? Do you exercise enough? Do you frequent places with polluted air? Do you pollute your own air?

Water Do you drink enough water? Do you drink pure water? Do you drink high energy water? Do you drink tap water?

Food Do you eat fresh food? Do you eat whole food? Do you eat a large variety of food? Do you eat processed food? Do you eat fast food? Do you eat snack food? Do you eat junk food? Does your food contain all the nutrients you need?

Beverages Do you drink coffee? Do you drink colas? Do you drink sodas? Do you drink tea? Do you drink beer? Do you drink wine? Do you drink liquor? Do you drink milk? Do your beverages contain any nutrients?

Ideas Do you read the Bible daily? Do you attend church regularly? What TV programs do you watch? What movies do you see? What music do you listen to? What books and magazines do you read? Do you make sure your counselors (doc tor, lawyer, etc.) are Godly? Do you take advice from worldly people?

People Why do you think Scriptural warnings against sexual promiscuity are so frequent and forceful?—Germs? Yes. Certainly, sexually transmitted disease is rampant and potentially deadly (AIDS, syphilis, etc.) Do you think there is more to it than that?

Every time something bad goes into us it weakens us a little bit. Every time something good goes into us we gain a little bit of strength. **Our health is where it's at because of the thousands of 'little bits' that we take in every day. A little bit does make a difference.** Please consider changing, for the better, a little bit every day.

Our physical health is not very important when compared to all of eternity. In fact, our entire life on earth doesn't seem very important when compared to eternity, except that the decisions we make here will determine where we spend eternity. For those who decide to do things God's way, eternal life with Him is your overwhelmingly important reward, better health here and now is a nice little perk.

GLOSSARY

Alpha Radiation

There are three kinds of radiations emitted by radioactive material—Alpha, Beta and Gamma radiations. To measure the effect of radiations on biological (living) tissue a unit of measure called the rad is used. The effect of radiation on living tissue, however, depends not only on the energy deposited in the tissue but also the type of radiation. A rem., therefore, is a unit of a radiation dosage used to relate various kinds of radiations in terms of biological destruction. It equals the rad times a factor for the type of radiation called the relative biological effectiveness (RBE). Beta and Gamma radiations have an RBE of one. Alpha radiation has an RBE of 10.

Natural sources of Alpha radiation outside the body are relatively harmless, because the radiation is absorbed by the skin. An internal source, however, is very destructive.

Alveoli

Our lungs are filled with millions of tiny air sacs called alveoli. Pollutants, especially smoke, stimulate chemicals that break down the walls of these air sacs making it difficult for the oxygen and carbon dioxide exchange. Emphysema is one result.

Anabolic Steroids

Anabolic steroids are synthetic variants of the strongest male hormone testosterone. Anabolic means the build up or growth of tissues in the body. Anabolic steroids were first used by German troops during WWII to increase strength and aggressiveness. Russians administered anabolic steroids to male and

HEBREWS 10:26-27

If we deliberately keep on sinning after we receive the knowledge of the truth, no sacrifice for sin is left, but only a fearful expectation of judgment and of raging fire that will consume the enemies of God.

female athletes as early as 1952 and continued through 1976. It is reported that 59 Russian athletes who competed in the Olympic games from 1952 to 1976 died in their prime because of anabolic steroid use. Today, steroid use is at an all time high.

Aneurysms

An aneurysm is an abnormal swelling in a weakened arterial wall. When blood flows through the effected area, the artery bulges and may rupture.

Angina Pectoris

Pain in the center of the chest caused by exercise or stress indicating an inadequate supply of blood to the heart muscle.

Angioplasty

Any procedure used to widen the opening of an artery that is narrowed by atherosclerotic disease.

Angiotoxic

Any substance that has an adverse effect on the inside of an artery wall.

Antibiotics

Drugs composed of extracts of living organisms, such as molds, which have the ability to destroy bacteria. Many antibiotics are no longer effective because bacteria have become resistant. Bacteria become resistant by changing a small portion of their DNA called a plasmid. These bacteria will even share the plasmid with other bacteria, thus producing a large population of bacteria that can resist a wide range of antibiotics.

Antioxidant

Antioxidants are nutrients that are capable of protecting our cells from uncontrolled free radical damage. The term oxidation has come to mean any free radical activity, not just the activity of oxygen.

Atherosclerosis

A degenerative disease of the arteries in which

fatty plaques build up, limiting blood flow and encouraging blood clot formation.

Atomism

Throughout all of history there has been an ongoing controversy of whether or not the human body has the innate ability to heal, repair and maintain itself. In ancient Greece the term Atomism defined the school of thought against our body's natural healing powers. The opposite of Vitalism.

Atrophy

The withering of an organ, a gland, muscle, etc. that had been fully developed, usually caused by lack of use, or substitution.

Autointoxication

A poisoned state brought on by the body's inability to rid itself of wastes, usually through the colon.

Autolysis

The tearing down or self-digestion of tissue as when the powerful enzymes of the lysosome organelle disposes of its host cell when the cell is worn out.

Autonomic Nervous System

That part of the central nervous system that controls unconscious functions like digestion and heart rate.

Calories

A calorie is a measure of heat energy. In common usage it refers to the energy value of a particular food.

CAMP (Cyclic Adenosine Monophosphate)

CAMP is a chemical found in most cells. When it is in excess in immune cells, it inhibits the immune response of that cell.

Carbohydrates

Carbohydrates are the preferred source of energy for our body. They break down into glucose which is our body's main fuel.

Carbohydrates are formed in growing plants through the process of photosynthesis. During this process the plant captures energy from the sun and converts it to chemical energy which all animal life must use for its very existence.

Cellulose

Cellulose is an insoluble dietary fiber which performs many health promoting functions like binding with fat and cholesterol and carrying it out of the body.

Cerebral Cortex

The outer part of the cerebrum made up of gray matter and white matter. This is the seat of our intellect and our memory. This is the thinking part of our brain.

Chemical Imbalance

If a person were in perfect health and perfect peace, he would have no chemical imbalances in his body. We are taught that a perfect state will not be achieved this side of glory.

In the vernacular, it refers to any dis-ease physical or mental caused by either an excess or deficiency of any active body chemical such as enzymes, hormones, neurotransmitters, etc.

Coenzymes

Any nutrient that is required to assist cellular enzymes in the production of active body chemicals. Many vitamins have coenzyme activity.

Coronary Thrombosis

Thrombosis refers to the process of blood clotting. When plaque builds up on the inside of an artery that feeds the heart muscle, platelets accumulate at the site and release chemicals that start the blood clotting process. As the clot enlarges, it cuts off the flow of blood to the heart muscle and can bring on a heart attack.

Corticoids

Corticoids are hormones produced in the adrenal glands. They affect our stress response, our metabolic rate, our blood sugar level, the way we use minerals and many other processes.

Cortisol

Cortisol is a steroid hormone produced in the middle layer of our adrenal cortex. It helps control our body's utilization of fat, carbohydrate, protein and minerals.

Courageous

One of the attributes of Saints.

Creative

One of the attributes of Saints.

Detoxify

To detoxify is to purify or render harmless (non-toxic) any harmful (toxic) substance. The liver is responsible for the majority of detoxification for the body.

Diaphragm

The dome shaped muscle separating the abdominal cavity from the chest cavity. As the diaphragm contracts it flattens out, increasing the size of the chest. We call this breathing.

Endorphin

Endorphin is a morphine-like, narcotic, chemical produced in times of stress, pain, etc.

Enzymes

Enzymes are proteins that cause chemical reactions to occur. Enzymes affect every part and function of our body like; production of vital body chemicals, digestion, immune response, detoxification, reproduction, nerve flow, etc.

Ethanol

Ethanol is the kind of alcohol found in beer, wine, and liquor. Also called ethyl alcohol.

Faithful

One of the attributes of Saints.

Fiber

Dietary fiber is the indigestible part of food plants. It aids in the passage of food through the digestive system and gives bulk to feces allowing proper elimination. Fiber controls the absorption of fat, sugar, cholesterol and other things. It is credited with lowering the risk of colon cancer.

Formaldehyde

Formaldehyde is an antiseptic used for cleaning and disinfecting. It is also used to preserve tissues that have been removed.

Formic Acid

Ant bite poison.

Free Radical

Any substance that displaces (steals) an electron from another molecule. Also known as oxidation.

Gene

Each gene is a specific part of a chromosome, made up of a section of DNA (deoxyribonucleic acid) and controls the production of a specific protein (enzyme).

Glucose

A sugar used by the body to make energy.

Glycogen

Glycogen is a polysaccharide or complex carbohydrate that is stored by the body in the liver and muscle tissue and used as a source of fuel in the production of energy.

Goal Oriented

One of the attributes of Saints.

Gram

A gram is the basic unit of weight in the metric system. Fifteen drops of water weigh about one gram.

Hippocampus

A part of the brain that is a center for learning and memory.

Homeostasis

Those processes that maintain balance in our body in the face of challenge.

Hopeful

One of the attributes of Saints.

Hormones

Hormones are chemicals produced by the eight endocrine glands of our body. They provide chemical instructions and communication within the body.

Hypothalamus

This is the part of our brain where the hormonal and nervous systems of our body interact.

Iatrogenic

A word used in medical literature that means cause by a doctor or medical procedure.

Insoluble

Insoluble literally means incapable of being dissolved. Used here as a class or category of dietary fiber.

Ion

An atom having either a negative or positive charge.

Isolate

As used in our discussion an isolate is any nutrient that has been manufactured in a laboratory (synthetic) or removed from its original food source.

Isomer

This refers to chemicals that have the same percentage of composition but are different in physical properties or are arranged differently in three dimensional space.

Isotopes

An element or compound having the same atomic number as another element or compound but a different atomic weight. Radioactive isotopes give off rays during spontaneous decomposition.

Joyful

One of the attributes of Saints.

Lactobacteria

Used in our discussion in the generic sense. Includes all helpful bacteria in the intestinal tract.

Lecithin

A group of compounds containing a high percentage of phosphorus and fatty substances. While lecithin is not a whole food, it is not an isolate either.

Limbic System

Several parts of our brain that work together and helps our involuntary body functions. It is also the seat of our emotions and sense of smell.

Loving

One of the attributes of Saints. Love is patient, kind, NOT envious, NOT boastful, NOT proud, NOT rude, NOT self-seeking, NOT easily angered, keeps no record of wrongs, NOT evil, but truthful, protective, trusting, hopeful and has perseverance.

Lymphocyte

A white blood cell that is part of our immune system. It helps control viruses and cancer, among other things.

Methanol

Also called methyl alcohol or wood alcohol. It is a poison that can cause blindness and death.

Mitochondrion

The cellular organelle where energy is produced.

Myocardial Infarction

Myocardial infarction commonly called a heart attack, occurs when a coronary artery is blocked, shutting off the blood supply to the heart muscle. The effected tissue dies from lack of oxygen.

Neuron

A nerve cell including the long fibers protruding from it.

Neurotoxin

A poison which affects nerve tissue. For example, the infantile paralysis virus contains a very powerful neurotoxin.

Neurotransmitter

For a nerve cell to "fire," the electrical charge on the interior of the cell must change from negative to positive. The nerve impulse then travels down the nerve to the synaptic knob where it causes chemicals to stimulate a target cell. These chemicals are neurotransmitters.

Norepinephrine

A hormone produced in the adrenal medulla which controls heart rate and blood pressure. As a drug, norepinephrine is used during surgery when blood pressure drops too low.

Nosology

The science of the classification of diseases.

Omnipresent

Present in all places at the same time. Only God is omnipresent.

Opiates

A class of narcotic drugs given mostly for pain relief. Morphine, codeine, heroine and demerol are all opiates.

Oxidation

We can define oxidation as the part of an oxidation-reduction reaction in which there is a loss of electrons by a species. Originally, oxidation simply meant a chemical combination with oxygen. The term was later broadened to include similar reactions.

Pandemic

A disease affecting an entire state or country or other large area in epidemic proportions.

Parasympathetic

That part of the autonomic nervous system which supplies nerves for the general purpose of restoring energy to the body.

Peaceful

One of the attributes of Saints.

Persevering

One of the attributes of Saints.

Pharmakia

This is the Greek word John used in Revelation 18:23. According to Vine's Expository Dictionary of Old and New Testament Words it "primarily signified the use of medicine, drugs, spells; then poisoning; then, sorcery." The only other place it is used in the Bible is in Revelation 9:21, translated 'magic arts' in the NIV.

Phytonutrient

Little understood class of chemicals in plant foods that have very beneficial effects on human health.

Placebo

A medicine having no active ingredient given to please or calm a patient, or fool a test group into believing they are receiving a medication.

Polonium-210

A radioactive substance found in high concentrations in tobacco that gives off the harmful Alpha radiation.

Portal Vein System

A network of blood vessels in the abdomen that pick up the results of digestion in the stomach, small intestines, colon, etc. and carries them to the liver.

Positive

One of the attributes of Saints.

Prosperous

One of the attributes of Saints. Originally prosperous meant "toward hope." The opposite of prosperous is despair.

Prostaglandins

A group of fatty acids made by the body that act a lot like hormones. They are usually made and used by the same tissue. They are important in circulation, immune response, kidney function and other ways.

Psychoactive

Drugs or other chemicals that have a profound affect on our thinking or mental processes.

Purposeful

One of the attributes of Saints.

Radioactive

Refers to any substance which emits radiant energy in the form of Alpha, Beta or Gamma rays or particles.

Radon

A radioactive gas given off by radium as it disintegrates.

Regeneration

The principal of natural healing philosophy which believes the human body has the ability to heal itself when given adequate nutrition and a poison free environment.

Ritalin

Ritalin is a central nervous system stimulant used primarily in children with Attention Deficit Disorders.

Saccharide

The basic unit that makes up carbohydrates.

Scientific Method

As used in our discussion, it is the accepted process by which a substance is proven safe and effective for healing in humans. Everything that does not meet this standard is, therefore, unproven and fraudulent.

Solar Plexus

A nerve center in the upper abdomen supplying nerves to the abdominal organs.

Soluble

Capable of dissolving. Used in our discussion as a class of dietary fiber.

Soul

The soul is that part of a person that is mental and emotional. It's the seat of a person's will and morality. It is different from the body and different from the Spirit.

Stevioside

It is that part of the stevia plant that tastes sweet.

Stimulus

Anything that results in a reaction.

Sucrose

Sucrose is simply the chemical name of refined sugar.

Sympathetic

That part of the autonomic nervous system which supplies nerves for the general purpose of expending energy.

Synergy

The cooperative action between two or more chemicals, nutrients, glands, etc. where the result is greater than the combined effects of each working individually.

Synthetic

Man made—not made by nature.

The Second Law of Thermodynamics

There are many aspects to this natural law. The one you need to understand is that without the addition of energy all processes move from order to disorder.

Thalamus

A mass of gray matter in the brain that receives and coordinates sensory information.

Ultraviolet

Ultraviolet light is invisible to the human eye. Most of the sun's ultraviolet light is absorbed by atoms in the upper atmosphere. That's good because large quantities are harmful. The ozone shield, that is in so much controversy these days, converts ultraviolet to infrared thereby warming the atmosphere.

Our bodies protect themselves from too much ultraviolet radiation by producing the skin pigment melanin. That, of course, is what gives us a suntan. Ultraviolet rays won't penetrate glass, so quartz lamps are used in those tanning salons you might frequent. By the way, those salons are probably not really a good idea.

Unconstitutional

Any law or act that is not in agreement with the principles laid down in the Constitution of the United States. Controversies arise over the interpretation of those principles.

Victorious

One of the attributes of Saints.

Visionary

One of the attributes of Saints.

Vitalism

Throughout all of history there has been an ongoing controversy of whether or not the human body has the innate ability to heal, repair and maintain itself. In ancient Greece the term Vitalism defined the school of thought that upheld our body's natural healing powers. The opposite of Atomism.

Referral Request

Virtually everyone knows people who are experiencing health challenges.

If you know people who you think would benefit by reading *Good Health God's Way*, and if you believe those people would apply Scriptural principles in their lives, and you would like us to send them a brochure and order form, simply tell us who they are.

Please make sure the address is accurate and complete.

Name ______________________________

Address ______________________________

City ____________________ State ___ Zip ________

Name ______________________________

Address ______________________________

City ____________________ State ___ Zip ________

Name ______________________________

Address ______________________________

City ____________________ State ___ Zip ________

If you would like us to enclose a personal note of recommendation and encouragement for you, we will be happy to do so.

My name is: ______________________________

Mail to: **Scriptural Nutrition Press**
P.O. Box 3085
Spring Hill, FL. 34611

ORDER FORM

Good Health God's Way may be ordered directly from the publisher. Groups, organizations or individuals ordering in volume shall receive the following discounts:

1-2:	$16.95 ea. + $3.00 ea. S&H
3-6:	$12.71 ea. + $2.25 ea. S&H (a 25% discount)
7-10:	$10.17 ea. + $1.80 ea. S&H (a 40% discount)
11 or More:	$ 8.48 ea. + $1.50 ea. S&H (a 50% discount)

Please send me the following:

Quantity		Unit Price	Total
	Good Health God's Way		
		Sub Total	
		Shipping and Handling $_______ per Book (see above)	
		Florida Residents, Add 6% Sales Tax	
		GRAND TOTAL	

Make check payable to: Scriptural Nutrition Press
P.O. Box 3085
Dept. 10
Spring Hill, FL. 34611

Please send my order to the following:

Name: ______________________________

Address: ______________________________

City: ____________________ **State:** ____ **Zip:** __________

Please allow 2-4 weeks for delivery

ALL DAY SEMINAR

If you agree with the principles and concepts presented in *Good Health God's Way* and would like Mr. Boyll to come to your area and present a one day seminar for your group or congregation, contact:

Scriptural Nutrition Press
P.O. Box 3085
Spring Hill, FL. 34611
Tel. 352-684-6087
Fax 352-688-6058